Yoga for Holistic Healing

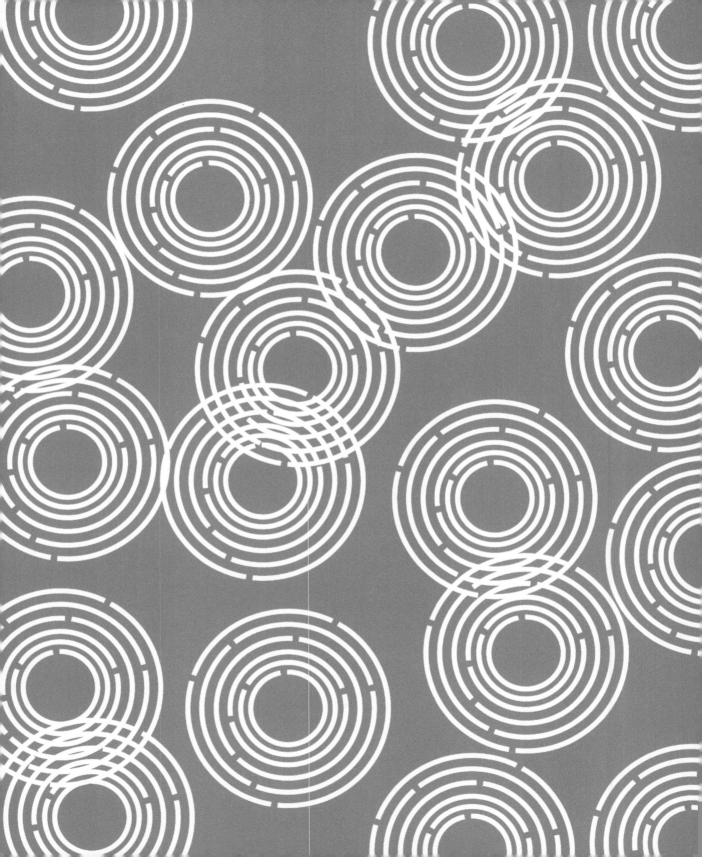

Yoga for Holistic Healing

Poses & Sequences for Pain and Stress Relief

Bonnie Golden , MEd, E-RYT

Illustrations by Charlie Layton

ROCKRIDGE PRESS

For general information on our other products and services or to obtain technical
support, please contact our Customer Care Department within the United States at
(866) 744-2665, or outside the United States at (510) 253-0500.

Rockridge Press publishes its books in a variety of electronic and print formats. Some
content that appears in print may not be available in electronic books, and vice versa.

Interior & Cover Designer: Erin Yeung
Art Producer: Karen Williams
Editor: Pippa White and Claire Yee
Production Editor: Rachel Taenzler
Illustration © 2020 Charlie Layton. Author photo courtesy of © Teresa Castro Photography.

ISBN: Print 978-1-64152-339-4 | eBook 978-1-64152-340-0
R0

To Norm

For your love, support in every way,
and for laughter

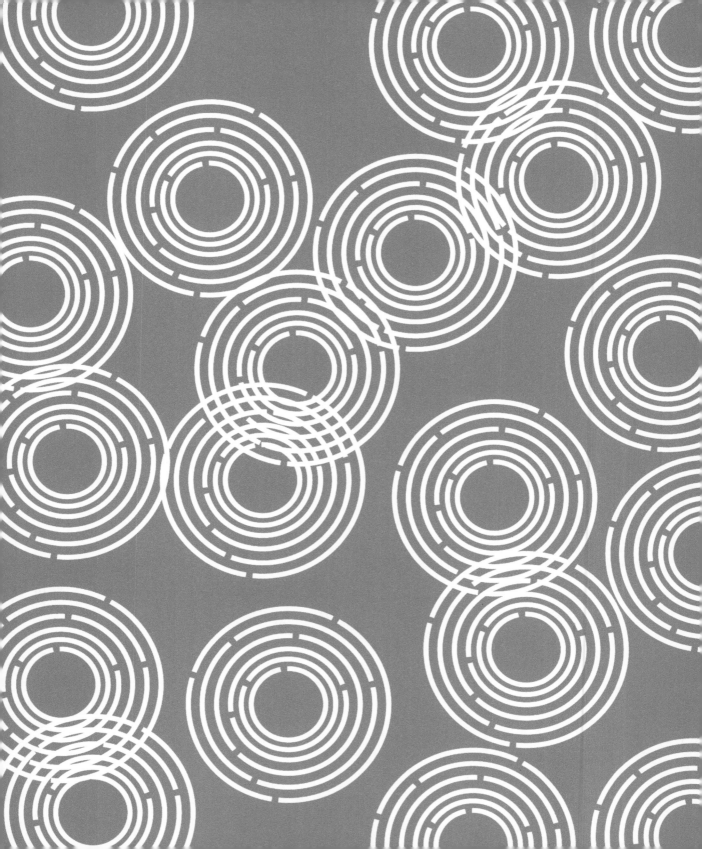

Contents

Introduction

Welcome as we embark together on this healing yoga journey! Yoga has supported my wellness and recovery through various health challenges; I hope you will be similarly supported by the practices in this book. I was first drawn to the meditative aspects of yoga through my musical heroes, the Beatles. At first, I had no idea how to meditate and no one to teach me. I attempted to practice yoga poses along with Lilias Folan on television, but I didn't have a clear sense of how to move my body. Eventually, I became a professional counselor and college faculty member. I began sharing yoga movements and breathing to help my students manage the physical and emotional symptoms of stress. As my yoga curiosity increased, I watched more practice videos, devoured yoga books recommended by friends around the country, and participated in formal yoga teacher training with world-renowned teachers, such as Baxter Bell, Tias Little, and Jill Miller.

Yoga also helped me manage my own stress—it was (and is) crucial to my mental equanimity as well as my physical self-care. I have suffered from frozen shoulder, sacroiliac dysfunction, and cough variant asthma. If it weren't for my holistic yoga practice, I know these disorders would have defined many of my days. Even when I'm not experiencing lower-back or shoulder pain, the stress-reducing and preventive benefits of yoga provide low-cost relief when my life gets too hectic.

In 2008, I transitioned to teaching yoga full time. I've deepened my learning and practice and guided thousands of students of all ages, conditions, and abilities.

All of it has come down to this message: I want *you* to practice *your* yoga!

Let me explain. When my students arrive to class or private sessions, they already have a variety of preconceived notions and diverse histories with yoga. Their yoga experiences range from watching YouTube videos to attending classes that were too fast, too hot, or too slow. Some of my students thought their bodies were not meant for yoga, that yoga was only for the young, slim, and flexible, or that their minds were too lively and scattered to take a class. Even so, something positive and healing drew them to try yoga again. Regardless of your background, the practices in this book will support you in practicing your healing yoga!

It's common for physicians, physical therapists, or counselors to recommend yoga to enhance holistic healing or manage a condition. Yoga provides a proven mechanism to address the multidimensional aspects of healing and pain relief. With the help of the poses and sequences in this book, you'll learn that one of the keys to harnessing the healing effects of yoga is connecting the breath, the mind, and the physical movements. As you go through the different sequences, you'll find that yoga practice is more effective than the sum of its parts.

This book is a complement to traditional health care and will empower and support you to participate in your health. You'll have the flexibility to pace yourself, repeat a sequence several times at your own speed instead of at the pace of a video or a class, and practice anytime. You may have a regular class you enjoy attending, but a current condition or injury is making it difficult to participate. This book can be your practice companion for any situation. If you are working with a medical professional, share this book so your provider knows you are doing this complementary practice. They may even have suggestions for particular poses or sequences.

Remember, it's *your* yoga!

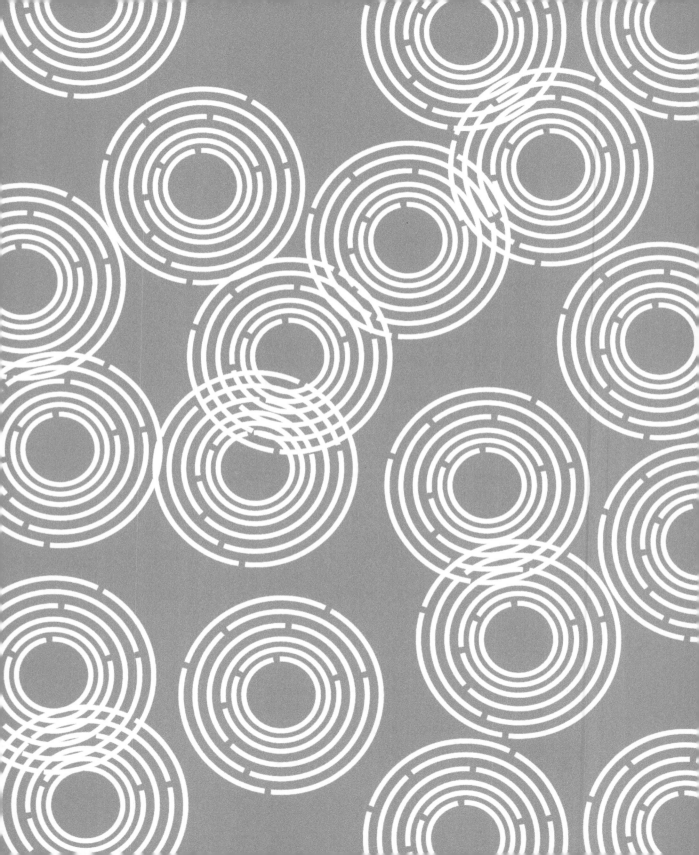

CHAPTER ONE

Yoga and Your Body

Understanding the human body is an important aspect of healing through yoga. Educating yourself about your body helps you develop self-compassion, mindful awareness, and the empowerment to create a personalized healing experience. In this chapter, you'll explore the poses, grasp the simple coordination of breath with movements, and learn about the role the brain plays in yoga healing. Welcome to the journey!

What Is Yoga?

The root of the Sanskrit word "yoga" is the verb "yuj," which means "to yoke or harness." The concept of unification also originates from yuj; this gives us the definition of yoga: *the process of uniting the mind, body, and breath in a holistic experience for the health and well-being of the individual.* In the broader sense, the ultimate goal of yoga is self-realization.

The vast tradition of yoga offers many expressions, practices, and paths to holistic unity and self-realization for the yogi, and the paths are not mutually exclusive. In brief, the primary paths include:

Bhakti Yoga. This is also known as devotional yoga. Prayer (in any religious tradition), chanting, and worship are bhakti yoga expressions.

Karma Yoga. This type of yoga deals with selfless action in the world. You are practicing karma yoga when you give your time and energy as a volunteer or care for others at work or at home.

Jnana Yoga. Knowledge and wisdom are the hallmark characteristics of jnana yoga. Your energy is primarily geared toward self-knowledge through meditation and working with a wise teacher.

Raja Yoga. Referred to as the royal path of yoga, raja yoga is frequently interpreted to include the essential eight-fold path, which includes:

- **YAMAS:** our treatment of others and the planet on which we dwell

- **NIYAMAS:** self-discipline and guidelines for living with intention

- **ASANAS:** the physical postures of yoga

- **PRANAYAMA:** breathing practices

- **PRATYAHARA:** withdrawal from sensory inputs, such as sounds and sights, in order to turn our attention inward to the body, mind, and breath

- **DHARANA:** sole focus on a primary object, such as breath, mantra, or visualization

- **DHYANA:** meditation in all its forms

- **SAMADHI:** joy and connection to all

A yoga pose, or asana, is a shape created with our physical body for strength, flexibility, joint health, comfort in meditation, or relaxation. You can practice yoga poses in any relationship to gravity: standing, seated, on your back, on your belly, and in inverted postures. A yoga sequence, or vinyasa, is a series of poses practiced in a particular order based on intention and coordinated with the breath. As you continue to practice yoga, you will become more aware of your thoughts, feelings, and breath. The unity inherent in practicing yoga creates a wonderful mental and physical experience of healthy, vital flow.

The earliest found evidence of yoga dates to 2700 BC in the Saraswati Valley. Seals and fossils in that region revealed evidence of postural and breath practices, according to Dr. Ishwar V. Basavaraddi. It wasn't until 200–500 AD—when the sage Patanjali systemized and codified yoga through 195 short guidelines called sutras, meaning "threads"—that yoga became a written transmitted tradition. Each sutra is a rich learning tool, and most yoga schools and teachers include the study of *The Yoga Sutras of Patanjali* in their curriculum today. The eight limbs of yoga described on page 2 originate from this text.

In her review of 20th-century yoga, scholar Amy Vaughn notes that in 1893 Hindu monk Swami Vivekananda spoke about yoga philosophy at the Chicago Parliament of Religions. This event is widely acknowledged as the first formal introduction of yoga philosophy in the United States. Another key presentation took place in 1920 when Paramahansa Yogananda, a monk, yogi, and guru, spoke in Boston. Yogananda founded the famous ashram and gardens in Encinitas, California, and is the author of *Autobiography of a Yogi*, which is available in 50 languages. Throughout the mid to late 20th century, students of yogi Sri Krishnamacharya brought their various forms of yoga (see page 5) to America. These students included B. K. S. Iyengar, K. Pattabhi Jois, Krishnamacharya's son T. K. V. Desikachar, and Indra Devi, a westerner who opened a yoga studio in Hollywood. Throughout the 1960s and 1970s, Richard Hittleman and Lilias Folan taught yoga on television. The popularity of yoga as a healing holistic medium has steadily risen over the past several decades (see page 8).

The Yoga Used in This Book

I have a simple yoga philosophy: Yoga equals awareness. The yoga practices in this book reflect my teaching and emphasize becoming healthy, self-aware, and empowered. This awareness includes the insight that consistently practicing poses in combination with breathing and thought awareness will promote healing, alleviate pain and mental suffering, and support us in our day-to-day life challenges. Yoga helps us be more in tune with our environment. We can discern if we are in situations that nurture us or detract from our health.

If we are moving or stretching our bodies without awareness of our mind and breath, we might enjoy the resulting feelings, but we aren't using the powerful integration of the mind/body/breath that is the crux of yoga and yoga healing. Yoga is self-empowering. The practice can simultaneously restore feelings of vitality, strength, and peace.

This book offers poses and sequences that are alignment-informed, breath-supported, and available in several variations. You'll hold some poses for several mindful breaths, and you'll move in and out of others while breathing in synchronization with the movements. Some will be a combination of both styles. I've been trained primarily in Iyengar, Viniyoga, Yin yoga, mindful meditation, and restorative yoga. I teach specialized classes and workshops about yoga for healthy aging, prenatal yoga, pelvic floor awareness, and Yin yoga. The poses and sequences in this book are from a combination of these yoga and contemplative styles, all inspired from my studies and practice in this wide variety of yoga and meditation traditions. The Most Common Types of Yoga explains each of the yoga styles in more detail.

Some sequences include props, such as blocks, to support or sense muscles, and straps that can help you inhabit poses by bringing more reach to your arms. You can also substitute household items for the props, such as bathrobe ties or neckties for straps, and thick books or tightly rolled towels for blocks.

The Most Common Types of Yoga

Depending on where you live, you might find that a few styles of yoga classes are dominant and others are not offered. Furthermore, the experience and style of the teacher will affect the character of a class. The most common yoga styles in the United States are:

Ashtanga. Ashtanga yoga is a vigorous yoga style, founded by Sri K. Pattabhi Jois, in which there is an emphasis on linking breath and movement. In a dedicated Ashtanga yoga class, students practice a series of postures called sun salutations and their variations. Increasingly challenging postures follow sun salutations and are categorized in three series: primary, intermediate, and advanced. According to a *Yoga International* interview with U.S. Ashtanga teacher Tim Miller, the primary series is therapeutic, building strength and joint flexibility. The intermediate series supports the breath flow, or prana, and the advanced sequences further stabilize the body and mind. Ashtanga classes are often referred to as vinyasa-style yoga. "Vinyasa" means to place in a prescribed order. However, vinyasa style can be applied to specific sequences in any yoga system.

Desikachar/Viniyoga. According to the American Viniyoga Institute, "viniyoga" refers to an approach that modifies yoga methods to the unique conditions, needs, and interests of each individual. Viniyoga was developed by Gary Kraftstow from the teachings of T. K. V. Desikachar of Madras, India. Viniyoga practitioners work one-on-one in a yoga therapy relationship. The practice emphasizes moving in and out of postures with the breath and then holding the asanas. It often includes the use of yoga tools such as chanting and mantras.

Hatha. According to yoga historian Amy Vaughn, author of *From the Vedas to Vinyasa*, the term "hatha" means "force" and is a combination of "ha" (sun) and "tha" (moon), signifying the balancing of opposites. It encompasses both physical and mental practices, such as posture, yogic breathing, focusing the mind, and meditative practices. Hatha yoga classes often have a slower pace and use all practices of yoga, from the physical to the meditative. However, most forms of yoga

continued

in the West can be called hatha if you are practicing postures, yogic breathing, and/or meditation.

Hot/Bikram. Hot yoga classes, a style originally popularized by Bikram Choudhury, are taught in a room heated up to 104°F. There are 26 postures taught in the same order, with breathing exercises at the beginning and end of each class. Many students who participate in hot yoga classes, whether Bikram style or simply in a hot room, report feeling more flexible, invigorated, and physically challenged. For other students, the heated room can result in adverse reactions, such as nausea and dehydration. According to a *Washington Post* review of hot yoga, if you have a preexisting condition, such as cardiovascular disease, back pain, asthma, diabetes, or are pregnant, other styles of yoga would be more suitable.

Iyengar. Iyengar yoga is named after its developer, B. K. S. Iyengar. In a dedicated Iyengar-style class, students practice a posture for extended periods, focusing primarily on physical alignment. There may not be many poses offered in a typical session, as optimal alignment and inner exploration of the body and breath are encouraged. One of the greatest gifts of Iyengar-style yoga is the use of modifications and props to make yoga accessible to all bodies and health conditions.

Kundalini. "Kundalini" means "coiled snake." Our untapped potential and energy is like a quiet snake located at the base of the spine. Kundalini yoga practices are said to awaken and uplift this latent energy to fulfill our life's purpose. In kundalini yoga classes, centuries-old yoga exercises called "kriyas" are practiced with vigorous breath practices, chanting, visualization, and meditation in a specific sequence. Kriyas are designed to produce desired effects, such as quieting or energizing the mind and body. According to the leaders of kundalini yoga, "kriya" means "work" or "action." Sikh master Yogi Bhajan brought Kundalini yoga to Canada and the United States, established the 3HO (Healthy, Happy, Holy Organization), and created ashrams in North America. Recently, promising research from the Alzheimer's Prevention

Organization has shown that the meditation chant kirtan kriya from Kundalini yoga reduces stress levels and increases activity in areas of the brain that are central to memory.

Restorative. Restorative yoga is a form of practice in which students are supported by props to cultivate relaxation and the down-regulation of stress in a dark, quiet, and safe space. Created by B. K. S. Iyengar, the style was popularized in the United States by his student Dr. Judith Lasater. Restorative yoga includes the use of bolsters and blankets to help practitioners feel supported. This style of yoga has a calming effect on the body, mind, and breath. Although some restorative poses are similar to yin poses, the intention differs. Restorative yoga's goal is complete relaxation and support, whereas yin poses are intended to put healthy stress on the deep connective tissues.

Sivananda. Sivananda yoga was founded by Swami Vishnudeva-nanda, one of the first Indian Yogis who came to the West, in 1957. His teacher was Swami Sivenanda. Vishnudevananda summarized the ancient wisdom of yoga in five principles or points that can be incorporated into daily life: asana, breath, relaxation, vegetarian diet, positive thinking, and meditation. Although there are some vigorous postures in the core physical practice, Sivananda classes can be modified. Sivananda yoga includes service to others, self-knowledge, and learning about Indian philosophy.

Yin. Yin yoga, which has been gaining popularity over the past 10 years, is a quiet practice that targets the health of connective tissues, including the fascia, ligaments, and joints. Poses are held for anywhere from two to five minutes to stimulate the deeper bodily tissues that can become stiff and inflexible. Yin yoga practice contrasts with yang practices, which are more active and muscular (such as Ashtanga or hot yoga). Yin poses target a particular area, such as the lower back, chest, or shoulders, to open over time and with stillness. There is a meditative quality to yin that can be challenging yet soothing. The primary figures in the popularization of Yin yoga in the United States are Paul Grilley, Sarah Powers, and Bernie Clark. It was originally founded by Paulie Zink.

Why Use Yoga as a Healing Medium?

According to the National Center for Complementary and Integrative Health (NCCIH), yoga is one of the top 10 complementary health approaches used in conjunction with conventional medicine to improve health and wellness in the United States. In fact, over a five-year period, a National Institutes of Health survey revealed an increase from 9.5 percent to 14.3 percent in yoga practice by adults. A recent Yoga Alliance and *Yoga Journal* study showed that the number of U.S. yoga practitioners has increased from 20.4 million to more than 36 million over the past seven years!

There are multiple benefits to choosing yoga as a healing tool, and the explosion in the number of yoga practitioners in the United States is a testament to this.

Most of us have an intuitive sense of what it means to heal. We've all had the experience of scraping our skin or perhaps breaking a bone. Eventually, these injuries get better. In a broader sense, according to a survey in the *Annals of Family Medicine*, healing can be considered a multidimensional path toward wholeness and personal growth, as well as an integration of the mind, body, and spirit.

As you practice yoga, you will experience that unique integration and healing of the physical, mental, and spiritual. Your practice will help improve strength, balance, flexibility, mindfulness, breathing, and more. Often within one practice session, my students observe a more integrated mental attitude and less physical pain. Yoga emphasizes mindful movement with simple breathing coordination. We move our large muscles and create hydration and circulation in our deep connective tissues. Simple joint-freeing postures reduce stiffness. Remaining quiet in certain poses allows gravity to unravel tension and stress in the tissues. I often quote the adage "Motion is your lotion." With mindful yogic movements, yoga can become your lotion.

For example: If you can, slowly raise your right arm up alongside your right ear; then, with the breath, move the arm sideways over your head and to the left. Keep breathing and stay tuned in to what you are physically experiencing. Do you notice an opening and stretch along the right side of the body to the top of your hip bone? If you repeat that movement with the left arm, the connective tissues, joints, and muscles on the sides, front, and back of, the body will lengthen. This simple demonstration shows that yoga practice has deeper and greater effects than the sum of the individual movements.

After enjoying these sequences several times a week, you will quickly notice a sense of inner peace and mindfulness in your daily life. Yoga is a wonderful way of reducing stress, managing distractions, and staying focused. On the practical side, yoga is portable—wherever you are, you have your yoga. For instance, you can breathe yogically to relieve the negative effects of stress on a long flight or when you are stuck in traffic. Yoga is low cost and needs minimal to no equipment. Yoga is time-tested, endorsed by practitioners, and scientifically proven. The science-backed medical benefits of yoga are highlighted on page 15. Evidence-based studies explain how yoga promotes the healing of specific conditions. Many of the practices in this book will address them.

Key Yoga Concepts to Help You Heal

Yoga tradition provides useful models for understanding your body, mind, and breath. As you practice the yoga routines in this book, think of the kosha model ("kosha" means "sheath" or "covering") as a helpful framework to address healing from a holistic yogic approach. The kosha model originated in an ancient yogic text called the *Taittiriya Upanishad*. The human being consists of five layers, or koshas: the physical body, the energy and breath body, the mind, the inner wisdom, and the bliss layer. Healing in one kosha will permeate healing in the other koshas. We can employ the interconnected kosha model when practicing the sequences in this book and be aware that our practice supports holistic yoga healing.

The Physical Body, or *Annamayakosha*

The annamayakosha is our physical body: "anna" (food) "maya" (consists of) kosha. To enhance health and healing, we need exercise and movement, water, and good eating practices. The poses (asanas) and sequences in chapters 2 and 3 directly address the physical well-being and healing of this kosha. Research has given us plenty of evidence on how yoga enhances our physical health. A review of comparison studies on yoga and exercise in the *Journal of Alternative and Complementary Medicine* demonstrates that in both healthy and diseased populations, yoga poses can be as effective as or better than traditional exercise in improving our health.

Our physical body consists of skin, bones, muscles, and a variety of internal systems of organs that coordinate and work together. A lesser-known part of our annamayakosha is fascia, a tissue that surrounds and connects all our body structures, providing support and protection. It includes sensory neurons and serves as a shock absorber. In *The Roll Model*, fascia expert Jill Miller uses an orange as an analogy. If you peel an orange, you will see a thick white coating under the orange skin. That coating is closest to our skin, like superficial fascia. The orange segments are held together by deep fascia, and the segments themselves have a light white coating of fascia. If we didn't have fascia providing structure, our body and its organs would have little shape and support.

We know that our fascia, and thus our body, can become stiff if we don't move. This is especially true when we are in pain and avoid movement completely. The poses and sequences in this book address stiff fascial connective tissue through mindful movement and allow the tissues to rehydrate.

The Energy/Breath Body, or *Pranamayakosha*

Prana is the universal life force that enlivens beings and spaces in this world, and pranamayakosha is our life-force body: "prana" (life force) "maya" (consists of) kosha. You can feel this kosha when paying attention to your breath. You will become more conscious of your breathing while practicing the sequences in this book. Pranayama, also known as breath regulation, is the fourth limb of yoga. Shallow breathing or hyperventilating likely indicates stress and anxiety, and sometimes we find that we're holding our breath. Slowing and softening the pace of our breathing, and breathing a little deeper into the belly, ribs, and back (360-degree breathing, see page 13) will provide stress release. Pranayama is as integral to yoga as breathing is to life. You can practice pranayama during asanas, but also anytime as a stand-alone practice to focus the mind as a pathway to meditation. Pranayama is a key connection to the nervous system: quieting, calming, balancing, or stimulating. See page 13 for yoga breathing instruction.

A recent analysis in the *Journal of Ayurveda and Integrative Medicine* of more than 1,400 studies demonstrates a preponderance of evidence of the positive effects of yoga breathing on clinical conditions and stress. The benefits of pranayama include reduced anxiety and depression, lowered or stabilized blood pressure, increased energy, relaxed muscles, decreased stress, and improved cardiorespiratory efficiency. Raising consciousness of and changing our breathing helps us manage stress levels and improve our physical and mental states. By consciously extending our exhales, we engage the relaxation response (parasympathetic system). When we concentrate our mind to breathe deeply, we decrease anxiety. Many conditions and diseases are directly related to or can be exacerbated by stress. Conscious breathing not only combats stress and its deleterious effects, it is also the foundation of many stress-management practices.

The physical postures of yoga support our breathing by expanding our capacity to increase diaphragmatic strength and flexibility, along with the accessory muscles of the breath. Posture, flexibility, and strength can affect our ability to breathe optimally.

From the yogic perspective, pranayama connects us to the greater life force in the universe and to all other sentient beings, keeps us present and mindful, and is the pathway to meditation and self-realization.

The Mind, or *Manomayakosha*

Manomayakosha is the thinking mind, which consists of our thoughts, beliefs, and opinions: "manos" (mind) "maya" (consists of) kosha. Much of this kosha is mediated from the input of our five senses. Our self-talk, affirmations, mantras, and visualizations are created in the thinking mind. We learn many meditation techniques through observing this kosha. Manomayakosha is important to our logical thought capabilities as we educate ourselves about pain, the breath, and the mind (as described on page 17). When we understand our mind's relationship to pain, combined with the yoga movements and breath practices in this book, we enhance yoga healing.

Inner Wisdom, or *Vijnamayakosha*

When you are able to objectively observe your own thinking, responses, and feelings, you are enlisting the vijnamayakosha: "vijna" (wise/discriminating knowledge) "maya" (consists of) kosha. This kosha can be described as witness consciousness, or the seer. I often think of this part of ourselves as our inner teacher. Yoga master Erich Schiffman refers to it as the "helicopter mind," the part of us that can observe without judgment. Our inner-wisdom self helps us avoid knee-jerk reactions to stressful situations and people. When employing vijnamayakosha in the sequences, you can compassionately ask yourself, "Am I breathing?" or "Am I thinking healing thoughts?" or "Am I catastrophizing?"

Bliss Layer, or *Anandamayakosha*

This kosha is the deepest layer of our being: "ananda" (bliss) "maya" (consists of) kosha. It can be viewed as our inner light of love, joy, happiness, and our true self. Anandamayakosha is our unchanging pure sense of value as a human being. It can be obstructed by issues and challenges in the other koshas. As you practice yoga healing, you'll begin to experience inner contentment and an appreciation of the good in yourself simply because you are you.

Yoga Breathing

Our breath gives us life. We breathe even if we aren't paying any attention to our respiratory function. For centuries, the yoga tradition has provided many practices to harness and manage our breath's potential for different effects. The following are three pranayama techniques that will support you in your healing journey.

Breath Exploration and Awareness

You can start or end every practice session with the important step of being aware of your breath. Continue to pay attention to your breath throughout your sequence.

1. Lie on the floor with knees bent. If possible, place a pillow or other support under your head and neck. Otherwise, it's fine to practice seated. Your eyes can be open or closed.

2. Begin to notice where you feel your breathing. Is it in the nostrils, in the chest, or in the belly? Does your breath feel smooth, deep, or somewhere in between? From your inner teacher, observe your breathing without judging it. There's no right or wrong.

3. Now experiment with placing one hand below your navel and the other on your sternum. Can you feel if your breath resides in one area more than the other?

4. Continue for as long as you'd like. Notice if your mind settles and your physical tension changes. Bring this simple breath-awareness practice, the fact that you are alive and breathing, into your sequence and your day.

The 360-Degree Breath

This breath helps increase our breath capacity and potential by employing the accessory muscles of breathing, called the intercostals, that reside between the ribs. The 360-degree breath helps cultivate a sense

continued

of breath distribution to the front, sides, and back of the body. When we focus our mind on the length of our breath, we begin to calm and unwind. We change our relationship to pain by managing distracting thoughts and focusing on breath sensations.

1. Begin with breath exploration and awareness, lying on the floor with knees bent.

2. Place a yoga block, a book, or a soft towel below your navel. If you are seated, lightly place your hands below your navel. Breathing through your nose, allow your breath to gently expand the belly as though filling a glass of water from the bottom up. Notice the belly fill on the inhale and recede toward the spine on the exhale. Think of your breath as long and slow. The prop or hands on your belly should rise with the inhale and relax back toward the spine on the exhale. If this is difficult because of a respiratory issue, stay calm and come back to the breath-awareness practice. Don't suck in the breath. Slow it down! Because of tight clothing, posture, or stress, it may take some practice to take what is often called a complete yoga breath. Be patient.

3. Once you feel comfortable with step 2, place your hands on either side of your ribs. Gently spread all your fingers except your thumb between the spaces of the ribs. The thumb rests toward the back body. Now begin long, slow, and deep complete yogic breaths, directing your breath into the muscles between the ribs, like an accordion expanding sideways. Can you feel the lateral expansion of the ribs on the inhale? Can you feel the contraction on the exhale? That is the coordinated result of the muscles of the diaphragm and the intercostals working together.

4. Take a few minutes before or after your sequence to harness the power of the 360-degree breath.

Lengthen Your Exhales for Calm

Lengthening the exhales is a tool to quiet our stress response and calm the nervous system. There is folk wisdom in the long sigh of relief!

1. Once you've established your long, slow, deep breath, begin to count the length of your breaths. The goal is for your exhales to eventually be about twice as long as your inhales. For example, inhale for a slow count of five (everyone's baseline breath capacity will differ), and exhale for a slow count of seven.

2. Repeat six times.

3. As your breath capacity increases over time with consistent practice, inhale for a count of five, and exhale for a count of eight.

4. With consistent yoga practice, you may be able to work toward a 1:2 ratio.

The Science-Backed Medical Benefits of Yoga

For many generations, direct and positive yoga experience has healed practitioners. Health care providers frequently recommend yoga to patients as a holistic complement to standard medical treatment. Evidence-based research now adds validation to this time-tested method for improving health, diminishing physical pain, and alleviating mental suffering. In fact, yoga physician Dr. Timothy McCall observes that the quality and quantity of scientific research proving yoga's healing properties has increased by more than 50 percent since 2010.

A recent study in the *Annals of Internal Medicine* shows that yoga is as effective as physical therapy for treating chronic lower-back pain. The 320 participants who practiced yoga were less likely to use pain medication than the control group, and they maintained their practice after the research concluded. The *Clinical Rehabilitation* journal recommends yoga as an accessible option for those who experience chronic neck pain.

Your brain can change as a result of regular yoga practice. Gray matter is uniquely correlated with pain tolerance, and recent research in *Cerebral Cortex* demonstrates that doing yoga increases gray matter volume in our brains.

Osteoarthritis is a common cause of pain in our joints. Research from the *Journal of Rheumatology* demonstrates that yoga practice helps individuals with arthritis safely increase physical activity. Participants in the study also experienced enhanced psychological and physical well-being. In other research, individuals with low bone density or osteoporosis improved bone-density measurements through practicing 12 yoga poses. As reported in *Topics in Geriatric Rehabilitation*, these poses improved balance ability and strength, and helped prevent painful falls.

To date, Dr. Timothy McCall has documented 117 health conditions helped by yoga, ranging from depression and anxiety to diabetes and cardiovascular disorders.

Yoga emphasizes the interrelationships of the mind, body, and breath. As you regularly follow the practices in this book, you will experience healthy side effects from the yogic whole-body connection. When you employ simple yogic breathing, the mind calms and your anxiety diminishes. The meditative, focusing tools of yoga will help you concentrate and reduce your worries. Your sleep will improve. Your muscular and joint-related aches and pains will diminish because you will learn to practice postural improvement and alignment. Yoga also strengthens your muscles because you use your body weight to practice many poses.

A meta-analysis in *Psychoneuroendocrinology* by Pascoe and colleagues highlights that yoga is a widely acknowledged and proven method to manage stress. Managing stress can reduce the occurrence of conditions such as cardiovascular disease, asthma, and gastrointestinal problems.

Our physical body is more than a set of disconnected parts. It is a system. In this book, you might find that a foot-pain sequence will include calf stretches, as many of the muscles of our feet originate above the foot. You might notice that lower-back stretches on your right side will release tightness in your left shoulder. The human body has fascia, or layers of connective tissue, under the skin that surround organs and muscles. It's like the connections in a spiderweb: if we move or stimulate one area of our body and its connective tissue, we often feel sensation or release in a totally different area. This is why it's important to practice the entire sequence on both sides of your body.

Meditation and Healing

Meditation is the practice of training the mind. Human attention is frequently scattered and drawn to external distractions. We also tend to become immersed in or even obsessed by internal thoughts, judgments, and stories. Our mind fluctuations often dwell in the past and the future, rather than in the present where the body and breath reside. Through mindfulness meditation and other forms of mind training that employ focusing tools such as our breath or a mantra, we will learn to direct our attention nonjudgmentally and compassionately to the precious present moment. Eventually, tension and stress begin to release through meditation, promoting our holistic healing. Meditation helps us remember we do not have to be defined by our pain. As we find our mind focusing on pain (and causing tension and stress), we can redirect our attention to the sensations of our breath.

Meditation practices have existed for thousands of years, and variations can be found in every spiritual or religious tradition. Herbert Benson's popular book *The Relaxation Response* demystifies meditation. Park and Han's comprehensive literature review in *The Journal of Alternative and Complementary Medicine* delineates findings that mindfulness meditation diminishes pain through multiple unique mechanisms, which is good news for the millions of chronic pain sufferers looking for narcotic-free, self-facilitated pain therapy. According to a review in *Current Opinion in Obstetrics & Gynecology*, mindfulness meditation has prominent effects on the psychological aspects of living with chronic pain, improving associated depression and the quality of life.

Understanding the Body and Identifying Pain Points

In order to understand pain and healing, it's important to first understand the human body. As you practice the poses and sequences in chapters 2 and 3, consult the illustrations on pages 19 and 20 and visualize the muscles and joints you are targeting for pain relief to make your practice more effective. As you see the larger landscape of the human body, use your movements, breath, and affirmations to envision healing in specific areas, harnessing the power of the body, mind, and breath.

I've divided the muscles into six general regions: head and neck; shoulders, arms, wrists, and hands; chests, abs, and back; hips, glutes, and pelvis; upper legs and knees; and calves, ankles, and feet. However, many groups correlate with one another. For example, the hamstrings are attached to the lower bones of the pelvis. If we have tightness in our hamstrings, it can affect our pelvis. You'll feel the connections in your body as you practice. Furthermore, as discussed on page 10, our body is also made up of ribbons of fascial connective tissue, as conceived by fascia expert Thomas Myers. You can see from the illustration of fascia on page 21 that the well-known plantar fascia under the soles of our feet is connected to the fascia all the way up the back of the body.

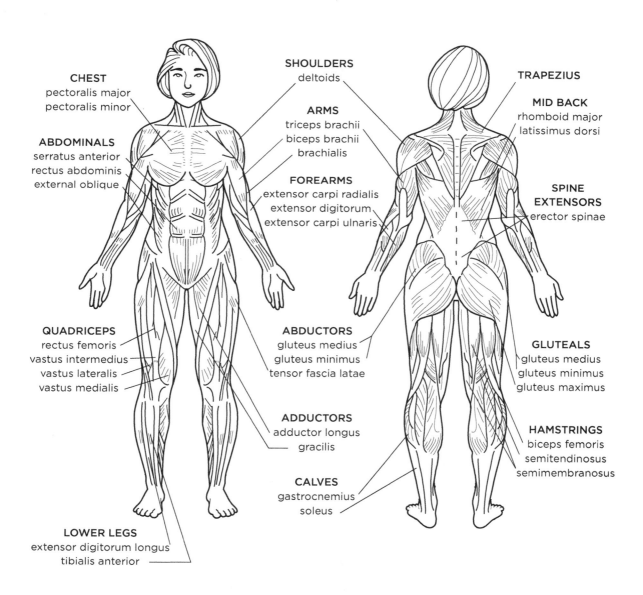

CHEST
pectoralis major
pectoralis minor

ABDOMINALS
serratus anterior
rectus abdominis
external oblique

SHOULDERS
deltoids

ARMS
triceps brachii
biceps brachii
brachialis

FOREARMS
extensor carpi radialis
extensor digitorum
extensor carpi ulnaris

TRAPEZIUS

MID BACK
rhomboid major
latissimus dorsi

**SPINE
EXTENSORS**
erector spinae

QUADRICEPS
rectus femoris
vastus intermedius
vastus lateralis
vastus medialis

ABDUCTORS
gluteus medius
gluteus minimus
tensor fascia latae

ADDUCTORS
adductor longus
gracilis

CALVES
gastrocnemius
soleus

GLUTEALS
gluteus medius
gluteus minimus
gluteus maximus

HAMSTRINGS
biceps femoris
semitendinosus
semimembranosus

LOWER LEGS
extensor digitorum longus
tibialis anterior

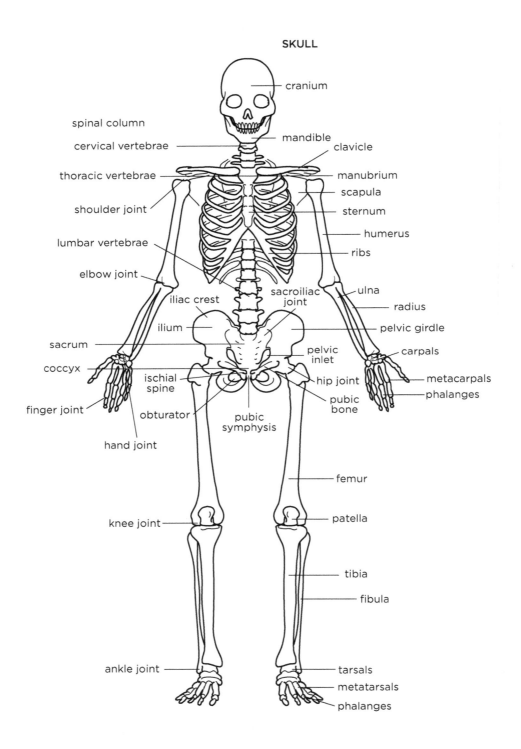

SKULL

cranium

spinal column

cervical vertebrae — mandible

thoracic vertebrae — clavicle

shoulder joint — manubrium

scapula

sternum

lumbar vertebrae — humerus

ribs

elbow joint

iliac crest — sacroiliac joint

ilium — ulna

sacrum — radius

coccyx — pelvic girdle

ischial spine — carpals

finger joint — pelvic inlet

obturator — hip joint

hand joint — pubic bone

pubic symphysis — metacarpals

phalanges

femur

knee joint — patella

tibia

fibula

ankle joint — tarsals

metatarsals

phalanges

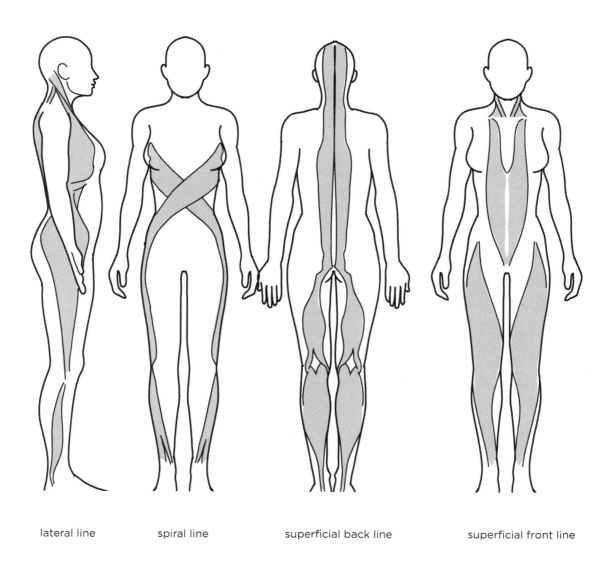

lateral line   spiral line   superficial back line   superficial front line

Fascia provide structure and stability to the body. These drawings illustrate the systemic
connectivity of our tissues. For example, you can see that a condition on the right side
of the body might be healed by bringing movement to the left side of the body.

HEAD AND NECK

- levator scapulae
- masseter
- neck extensors and flexors
- scalenes
- splenius capitis and cervicis
- sternocleidomastoid
- upper trapezius

SHOULDERS, ARMS, WRISTS, AND HANDS

- biceps brachii
- deltoids
- forearm flexors and extensors
- latissimus dorsi
- rhomboids
- rotator cuff muscles: supraspinatus, infraspinatus, teres minor, subscapularis
- serratus anterior

CHEST, ABS, AND BACK

- erector spinae
- external and internal obliques
- intercostals
- latissimus dorsi
- pectoralis major
- pectoralis minor

- quadratus lumborum
- rectus abdominus
- rhomboid major
- transverse abdominus
- trapezius

HIPS, GLUTES, AND PELVIS

- deep hip rotators (particularly piriformis)
- gluteus medius, gluteus maximus, gluteus minimus
- hip flexors
- iliopsoas
- pelvic floor
- quadratus lumborum

UPPER LEGS AND KNEES

- abductor group
- adductor group
- hamstring group
- iliotibial tract
- quadriceps group
- tensor fasciae latae

CALVES, ANKLES, AND FEET

- Achilles tendon
- flexors and extensors
- gastrocnemius
- plantar fascia
- soleus
- tibialis anterior

BONES AND JOINTS

- carpals, metacarpals, phalanges
- clavicle and scapula
- connective tissue lines
- femur
- humerus
- patella
- pelvis: sacrum, coccyx, ischial tuberosities, ilium, ischium
- radius and ulna
- ribs
- skull: cranium and mandible
- spinal column: cervical, thoracic, lumbar vertebrae
- sternum
- tarsals, metatarsals, phalanges
- tibia and fibula

Preparation

As you approach yoga from the perspective of holistic healing and prevention, the following guidelines will serve as important aspects of self-care, pain diminishment, and staying on the healing path. These recommendations mirror how I teach my live classes and private sessions. Although it is tempting to jump directly into the poses and sequences, take a few minutes to consider these points.

Curate Your Space

Environment can support our sense of safety or distract us as we practice. It's helpful to have a yoga sanctuary that will enhance attention to your practice. Don't worry about perfection. You don't need to have a separate room. You can select a corner of a room, or even a spot outdoors. Minimize distracting sounds or play quiet music. Leave the cell phone in another room and turn off the TV or computer. Be sure the temperature is comfortable and create pleasant lighting. Place a plant or a picture with a word such as "breathe" in your line of sight to invoke tranquility, peace, and joy. Ask other household members not to interrupt if you are unable to close a door. (If you have very young children, nap time might work best.) Whether you're practicing on a yoga mat, carpet, or chair, be sure you have plenty of room to move. For safety, make sure the chair legs are anchored directly to a wall or placed on a mat so they don't slip.

Wear What's Comfortable

Students often ask how to dress for yoga. There is no need to purchase new clothing. Simply wear garments in which you can breathe comfortably and move freely. Elastic-waist shorts or pants work well. You can even practice pajama yoga.

Choose Your Poses and Sequences

Think about how you are feeling physically and mentally today, and look for poses or sequences that will benefit areas that need attention. Do a visual review, rehearsing the sequence in your mind to help the mind and body connect to the movements during the actual practice. Be easy on yourself: There is always a learning curve when we are doing something new. Remember that you are worth the time, and regular practice will reap healthy benefits.

Create an Intention

After going to your practice space, allow for a few quiet transitional moments. Take a nice deep breath in and let it out. Sit down and mentally scan your body for residual tension you're holding. Let it go. Notice your thoughts. If your mind is drawn to stories from the past or plans for the future, simply escort your thoughts back to the present. Give your mind an anchor, such as the supportive mental affirmations or intentions provided, to stay focused. For example, "I now support my wellness through my practice" or "My yoga is holistically supporting my healing." Cultivate an attitude of self-care and self-compassion.

Breathe Consciously

As described on page 13, breath awareness is the key to stress and pain management. In yoga practice, you breathe consciously along with the movements. Yoga is different from stretching because of the emphasis on body, mind, and breath.

Long, slow, conscious breaths will support tension relief and unwind the stiffness, clenching, or guarding that happens in our muscles when we perceive pain. We often default to shallow breathing or even holding our breath as our brain associates a body part with pain. Pain science tells us that if we move gently, with our breath and our mental intention, into a point of tolerable discomfort, we begin to teach our brain to let go of movement fear and knee-jerk reaction to pain.

Tips for Success

As you embark on your journey of practicing healing yoga at home, here are a few more tips to help you make the most of your experience:

- Keep water handy. Even during light physical activity, it's important to stay hydrated.
- It is not necessary to have a completely empty stomach before yoga; however, to avoid feeling sluggish, wait 20 to 30 minutes after eating a large meal.
- Gather the recommended props ahead of time for the poses or sequence you've selected.
- For a holistic approach and well-rounded yoga experience, regularly change your selection of sequences and poses. For example, alternate sequences that focus on the upper and lower body, or alternate flexibility and strength practices.
- Remember that yoga is noncompetitive. Respect your current level of strength and flexibility and know you will accrue healing benefits with regular practice, regardless of your starting point.
- Work intelligently if you are in pain. Ask yourself if a particular movement is safe and if you will feel comfortable later. It's okay if there is a bit of tolerable discomfort.
- Pause and observe your physical feelings between sides or poses.
- Check in regularly with your breath. Your calm yogic breathing, as described on page 13, is a reliable sign of physical or mental ease. If you are breathing shallowly, holding your breath, or even hyperventilating, reflect on whether you need to stop the movement because it's truly dangerous and painful, or if you are in a habitual place of guarding yourself from pain.

How to Use This Book

This book is flexible and adaptable, just like yoga. I've designed the poses and sequences as a practical resource to allow you to individualize your yoga routine and meet your needs on any given day. You can address a specific concern or focus on general discomforts. You will also notice that some poses have variations, such as sitting rather than lying down on your mat.

Chapter 2 focuses on upper-body poses and sequences, and chapter 3 focuses on lower-body poses and sequences. Each chapter contains a selection of individual poses for each region of the body—for example, calves, ankles, and feet. However, remember that we are an interconnected system of body, mind, and breath. Poses that address back pain may include leg stretches or postural poses, as we know that tight hamstrings or less-than-optimal posture can directly contribute to back pain. The end of each chapter includes five focused sequences, each with a different theme:

Posture focus. Posture can be defined simply as how we position our body in everyday life as related to gravity: seated, standing, or lying down. Simple postural improvement can relieve back, pelvis, and shoulder pain. Postural improvement may also help expand our breath capacity.

Strength focus. Sometimes our muscles are weak because we neglect to challenge them appropriately, either as a result of avoiding pain or simply because we're not using them enough. Muscle weakness can also create pain in adjoining muscles. As compensating muscles take up the slack, they can become overused, sore, or tight. It is important to develop well-balanced strength so we can recover from pain and move confidently through life.

Flexibility focus. I like to think of flexibility as creating length and room in our tissues and joints. Tightness and guarding from various sources of stress, such as pain or the environment, can become habitual. It can affect our ability to walk up steps, reach for an item on a shelf, and even breathe well.

A little bit of everything. This sequence is well-rounded and derived from the upper- or lower-body chapter poses.

Unwind and de-stress. This series consists of yin and/or restorative poses (see page 7). You can practice it by itself or after any of the previous sequences. The sequence will release deep-tissue tightness and allow gravity and support to bring your body, mind, and breath to a calm state. For healing to occur, it is crucial for your yoga practice to be as much about being as doing.

You can combine the strength sequences from both chapters on one day or focus on the upper or lower body only, practicing several or all the sequences. Or maybe you want to focus only on shoulders. It's your yoga!

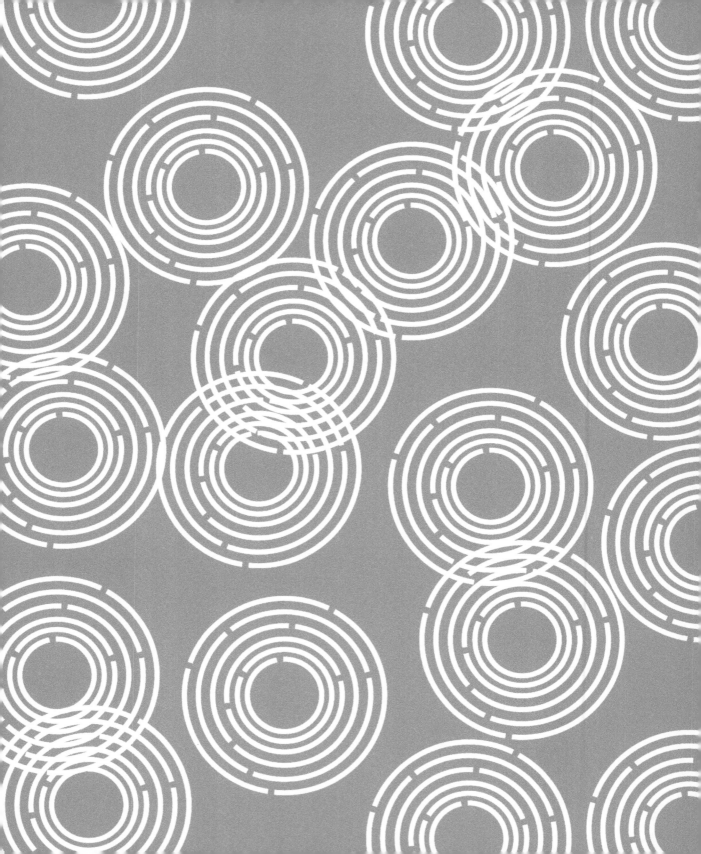

Upper-Body Poses and Sequences

The poses and sequences in this chapter will support your self-care, providing symptom relief and holistic healing for many conditions of the upper body. Your unique, individual, optimal spinal alignment is integral to the well-being of the three focus areas in this chapter: head and neck; shoulders, arms, wrists, and hands; and chest, torso, and back. Postural awareness, as described in Mountain Pose (see page 33), often contributes to the direct relief of aches or tightness in these areas and keeps you mindful, uplifted, and safe as you move in the practice. The position of our skull over our neck bones (cervical spine) or the position of our shoulders on our back can either exacerbate or help relieve lower-back pain. Additionally, factors such as persistent pain, physical stress from that pain, or even being bedridden can cause our muscles and connective tissues to accommodate after our pain or illness is long gone. We can become stiff and stuck in a protective posture. When you consider the fascia system (see page 10), you can see that a regular yoga practice on both sides of your body can provide relief to your entire system.

Remember to breathe consciously and follow the Preparation tips (see page 25) and Tips for Success (see page 27). If you have a flare-up of any condition, the restorative poses and simple breath practices are best.

Head and Neck

Bookmark this page! Each pose and sequence refers to different physical areas and muscle groups shown in this illustration.

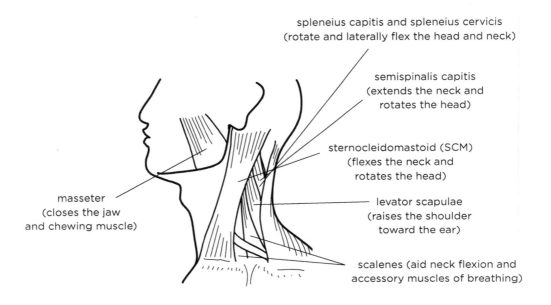

spleneius capitis and spleneius cervicis
(rotate and laterally flex the head and neck)

semispinalis capitis
(extends the neck and
rotates the head)

sternocleidomastoid (SCM)
(flexes the neck and
rotates the head)

masseter
(closes the jaw
and chewing muscle)

levator scapulae
(raises the shoulder
toward the ear)

scalenes (aid neck flexion and
accessory muscles of breathing)

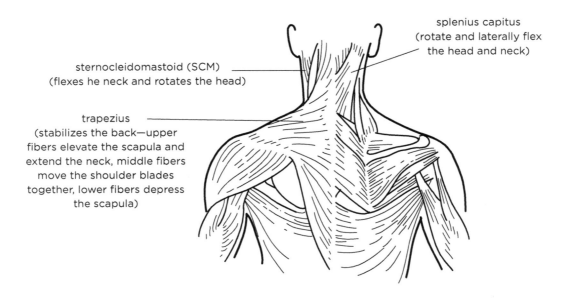

splenius capitus
(rotate and laterally flex
the head and neck)

sternocleidomastoid (SCM)
(flexes he neck and rotates the head)

trapezius
(stabilizes the back—upper
fibers elevate the scapula and
extend the neck, middle fibers
move the shoulder blades
together, lower fibers depress
the scapula)

MOUNTAIN POSE: POSTURAL AWARENESS WITH CHIN TUCKS

PHYSICAL AREAS TARGETED: all body systems from head to feet: levator scapulae, splenius capitis, semispinalis capitis, masseter, sternocleidomastoid, pectoral muscles in the chest (see page 68), rhomboids and trapezius in the back (see page 69), adductor group (see page 110), erector spinae (see page 69)

BODY AND MIND AREAS RELIEVED: neck pain, tight shoulders, slumped back

Mountain pose is the fundamental yoga pose to self-assess and embody healthy, healing postural and breathing patterns while modifying unhealthy habits. In this variation, you will notice and improve how the position of your head and neck affects the curves in your spine and pelvic alignment. You'll also strengthen your legs and improve where and how you stand on your feet. You'll feel a sense of mindfulness and poise when doing this pose. To help improve your posture, practice the chin tuck whenever you're working at your computer, driving, eating, or doing any other activity.

COMMON CONDITIONS ADDRESSED

- Back pain
- Decreased self-confidence
- Difficulty breathing
- Head-forward posture
- Hunching or humpback posture
- Lack of balance
- Pelvic pain
- Poor digestion
- Temporomandibular joint (TMJ) pain
- Tight or hunched shoulders
- Weak leg muscles, particularly the inner thighs

PROPS NEEDED: BLOCK (OPTIONAL)

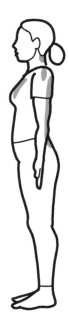

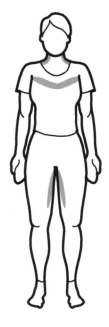

SIDE VIEW:
Earlobe over shoulder,
shoulder aligned with hip,
anklebone aligned with hip bone.

FRONT VIEW:
Toes forward,
chin level with floor,
bottom ribs over top of pelvis.

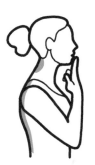

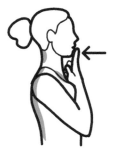

1. Stand with your feet hip distance apart, toes and palms forward, arms at your sides.

2. Slowly sway on your feet—left and right, forward and back. Notice how you bear weight on your feet. Do you apply more pressure on the inner or outer arch, or favor a heel or toe?

3. Adjust by placing slightly more weight on your heels, then the base of your big toes, and finally the base of your little toes. Feel all your toes connected to the earth. Spread them out for an enhanced base of support.

4. Engage the muscles of the legs without gripping them. If you'd like, place a block between your inner thighs. This will awaken the adductors, which are weak in many individuals.

5. Notice if your pelvis is shifting forward or back. Relax your shoulders away from your ears.

6. Gently engage the lower abdominal muscles.

7. Place one finger on your chin. Lengthen the neck forward as you press the chin into the finger, and then press the head back with your finger.

8. When your head is back, sense that your ears are even with your collarbones and feel the rear neck muscles engage. Keep breathing and repeat this "chicken neck" movement 5 or 6 times. Keep the jaw relaxed.

9. Release your finger and feel your poised mountain pose. Imagine making more room for your internal organs to do their job, especially the respiratory and digestive systems, as your entire spine lengthens.

10. Whenever you catch yourself in head-forward posture while sitting or standing, bring your finger to your chin and note the poise transmitted throughout your being.

- Using a mirror for a front view of your body, imagine a dotted line down the middle of it, and see if you can envision balancing your left and right sides symmetrically. Imagine an internal alignment, brain over heart over pelvis.

- Have someone take your picture for side-view alignment. Is your head thrusting forward? Can you align your ears with your collarbones?

- Don't thrust your chest (military posture).

MODIFICATIONS

- Bring your palms together at the heart. Breathe and pause as a standing meditation.

- Float your arms over the head alongside the ears, palms toward each other, for a full-body lengthening.

- Practice seated Mountain Pose to make sure you aren't habitually jutting your chin forward. Stack your knees over your ankles, ribs over hips, and head over neck. Avoid sitting on the tailbone, which tends to round the spine.

NECK ROTATIONS WITH OPTIONAL MANUAL TRACTION

PHYSICAL AREAS TARGETED: head and neck muscles, sternocleidomastoid, scalenes, trapezius, levator scapulae

BODY AND MIND AREAS RELIEVED: stiff neck, upper back, shoulders, head, and spine

Everyday habitual healthy or unhealthy postures (walking, sitting, reading) will echo throughout the spine, from head to neck to back to hips to feet. One common unhealthy habit is a head-forward posture, which is exacerbated by peering down at phones and other technology. This "tech neck" position can destabilize neck muscles and ligaments from overstretching and muscle imbalances. When our neck and upper back are pulled forward by the head, the entire spine often rounds (flexes), possibly contributing to disc and bone-quality degeneration. The gentle neck rotations movement series will ameliorate stiffness and hydrate tissues to keep them healthy. Consult your health care provider before doing this pose if you are currently experiencing whiplash, herniated disc, arm numbness, or extreme osteoporosis.

COMMON CONDITIONS ADDRESSED

- Decreased postural integrity

- Difficulty breathing

- Shoulder tightness

- Stiff neck from everyday habits, such as carrying a purse or backpack or sleeping too long in one position

PROPS NEEDED: NONE

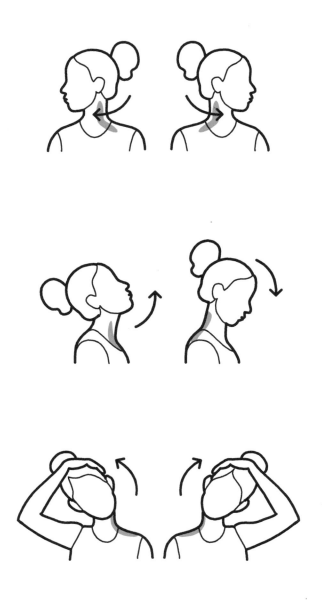

Breathe consciously and slowly in and out of each stretch.

1. Practice while standing in Mountain Pose (see page 33). Eyes can be open or closed throughout.

2. Keeping your head upright, inhale, then turn your head to left on the exhale. Consciously drop your right shoulder away from your right ear.

3. Inhale and turn your head back to the center, then exhale and turn your head to the right. Consciously drop your left shoulder away from your left ear.

4. Turn your head back to center. With a neutral head, tilt your chin up slightly to where the wall and ceiling meet until you feel lengthening in the neck and throat area.

5. Tilt your chin toward your chest and notice the lengthening and feeling of release at the back of the neck and upper back. Optional: Place the fingertips of your right or left hand on the back of your head and gently and slowly press your chin slightly more toward the chest.

6. Starting with a neutral head, bring your left ear toward your left shoulder. Avoid hiking the left shoulder up to the left ear. Keep gently dropping the right shoulder away from the right ear. Optional: Bring your left hand over your head and gently assist the stretch, providing further opening between the right ear and shoulder.

7. Starting with a neutral head, bring your right ear toward your right shoulder. Avoid hiking the right shoulder up to the right ear. Keep gently dropping the left shoulder away from the left ear. Optional: Bring your right hand over your head and gently assist the stretch, providing further opening between the left ear and shoulder.

TIPS

- Keep your jaw relaxed.

- Breathe consciously through each movement and stay in each position for 2 to 5 breaths.

- You might feel dizzy if you are not accustomed to turning your head. If so, back out of the movement and try again another time.

MODIFICATION

If standing is difficult for you today, you can practice this pose seated.

CAT/COW WITH NECK-FOCUSED TURTLE

PHYSICAL AREAS TARGETED: entire spine, with emphasis on: erector spinae (see page 69), upper trapezius (see page 68), levator scapulae, splenius capitis, splenius cervicis

BODY AND MIND AREAS RELIEVED: tightness in the chest, abdomen, and pelvis

The Cat/Cow pose gently flexes and extends the entire spine. It helps relieve tension in the neck, shoulders, mid back, and lower back. If you are obligated to be seated at work, or if you are traveling, you can practice seated Cat/Cow for ease in the entire spine. Simple breath coordination can flow easily through this movement. The front body receives opening and strength, particularly in the chest, shoulders, and abdomen. When you tune in to the physical and breathing rhythm of Cat/Cow, your mind begins to relax.

COMMON CONDITIONS ADDRESSED

- Back pain
- Decreased breath and movement coordination
- Decreased meditative focus
- Decreased pelvic awareness, particularly in pregnancy
- Decreased vitality in the internal organs
- Neck tightness
- Shoulder hunching

PROPS NEEDED: CHAIR (OPTIONAL)

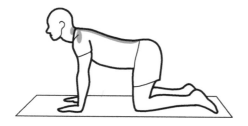 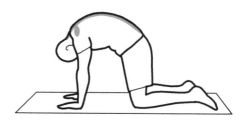

COW: Lengthen neck as shoulders and chest moves back, wrists under shoulders, knees under hips.
CAT: Mid back toward the sky, tailbone toward the earth.

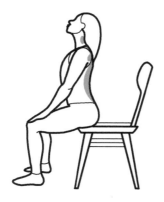 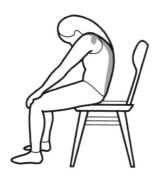

CHAIR VARIATION: Sit at the edge of the chair. Extend the spine without jutting your chin. On the inhale, lengthen your spine. On the exhale, round your spine.

1. Come to your hands and knees (Table Pose) on a mat. Align your wrists under your shoulders and your knees under your hip joints.

2. Press into the mat with all 10 fingers to take pressure off your wrists. Place additional padding under your knees, if desired.

3. Inhale and draw the chest back as you slide the shoulders away from the ears. Feel the neck lengthen like a turtle peeking out of its shell. Focus on elongating the entire spine, particularly the neck. There will be a mild arch in your back.

4. Exhale and round the mid back to the sky like a Halloween cat. Gently draw your chin toward your chest and your pubic bone toward the earth.

5. Alternate these movements as many times as you wish, staying for several breaths in either shape, or gently sway your hips to vary the sensations of the stretch.

TIPS

- Envision your neck as a natural extension of your spine. Make sure your chin isn't jutting toward the sky.

- Press your hands down into the floor, engaging your arm muscles to prevent your chest and belly from sagging.

- Sunbird (see page 76) and Downward-Facing Dog (see page 70) flow naturally from Cat/Cow. Feel free to rotate and stretch your wrists between the poses.

MODIFICATION

Seated Cat/Cow is an equally effective variation if coming to all fours is impractical. You can practice this variation anytime you are seated.

THREAD THE NEEDLE

PHYSICAL AREAS TARGETED: splenius capitis; splenius cervicis; upper trapezius; shoulder muscles, including infraspinatus, teres minor, rhomboids (see page 69)

BODY AND MIND AREAS RELIEVED: tense neck, tight shoulders, tight jaw, tight upper back

Thread the Needle is a versatile pose that provides tension release in the entire spine, particularly the upper back, neck, and shoulders. It is a calming pose that you can practice in the yin style to allow extra time for tension in the tissues to dissolve. Try holding one side at a time for 2 to 3 minutes, or moving dynamically in and out of the shape with your breath.

COMMON CONDITIONS ADDRESSED

- Decreased spinal mobility
- General spinal soreness
- Inner and outer body stress
- Neck pain
- Overactive brain
- Shoulder tension
- Upper back stiffness

PROPS NEEDED: PILLOW OR BLANKET (OPTIONAL)

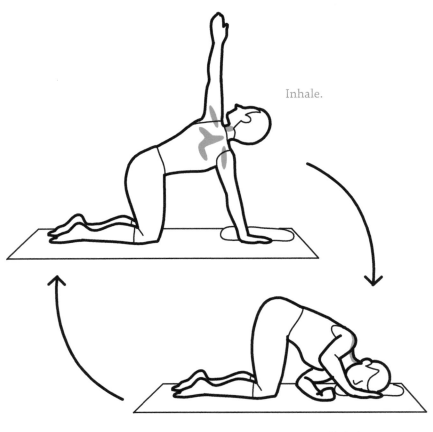

Inhale.

Exhale.

1. Come to your hands and knees (Table Pose) on a mat. Align your wrists under your shoulders and your knees under your hip joints.

2. As you press your right hand into the floor, inhale and raise the left arm up to the sky, enjoying the opening in the chest. You may stay in this shape for as many breaths as you'd like.

3. Sweep the left arm underneath the right arm as you bend the right elbow. Allow the back of your left shoulder and side of your head to rest on the floor, a pillow, or a blanket.

4. Keep the right palm on the floor with your elbow bent or stretch the arm straight in front on the floor to increase the opening on the right side of your body.

5. Remain here for 5 or 6 breaths.

6. Repeat, inhaling the right arm to the sky and threading it under the left.

7. Move into Cat/Cow with Neck-Focused Turtle (see page 40) or come to Child's Pose (see page 72).

TIPS

-   Keep your hips as level as possible.

-   As you feel release in the tissues, especially in the shoulder, you may be able to thread slightly deeper and move more onto your shoulder and upper back.

-   Come out of the pose if you feel tingling in the neck or arm.

MODIFICATIONS

-   Place a pillow or blanket under your head if getting your head to the floor is challenging.

-   Practice sitting on a chair if coming to Table Pose is impractical or difficult.

OPEN SEATED TWIST

PHYSICAL AREAS TARGETED: neck rotator muscles: scalenes, sternocleidomastoid, splenius capitis, splenius cervicis; back muscles: upper trapezius, erector spinae muscles (see page 69); chest muscles: pectoralis (see page 68); side-body muscles: obliques (see page 69)

BODY AND MIND AREAS RELIEVED: stiff back, tight chest, restricted breathing, lack of focus

Spinal twists are integral in yoga to maintain spinal range of motion and stimulate the muscles and bones along the back. The neck is part of the entire spine, and within a twist we can work mindfully to relieve neck tension. This gentle, open twist helps maintain our ability to turn our head, and it also helps relieve lower-back pain. It is safe to practice the open twist while pregnant, as the belly is not twisted. If you have spinal disc issues, please check with your health care provider before doing this pose.

COMMON CONDITIONS ADDRESSED

- Decreased focus, breath, awareness, and calm
- Lack of stimulation to internal organs
- Lower-back pain

- Osteoporosis (if practiced as instructed)
- Stress
- Tight neck

PROPS NEEDED: BLANKET(S) OR PILLOW (OPTIONAL), CHAIR (OPTIONAL)

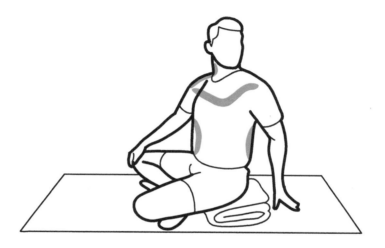

Keep the knees aligned with the pelvis by placing blankets under the hips. Keep the front hand on the same-side leg and maintain the lifted spine with relaxed shoulders.

1. Sit cross-legged on the floor so your knees are even or slightly lower than your hip joints. If your knees are higher or your lower back is rounding, sit on a folded blanket or pillow to elevate your hips and elongate the spine.

2. On an inhale, lengthen your spine and turn your belly, ribs, and chest to your left as you bring the right hand to the right leg. Once in the twist, lengthen your spine on the inhale, and feel your shoulders relax away from your ears on the exhale. Keep your chin level with the floor. Breathe in this manner for several breaths.

3. Explore your neck range of motion by slowly and slightly turning your chin or your gaze farther to the left.

4. If you feel pain at any point, inhale and unwind slightly, or slowly come out of the pose.

5. To exit the twist, inhale, lengthen your spine, and exhale to neutral.

6. Repeat the twist toward the right.

TIPS

- Think of the head turning last so the twist comes from the lower spine.

- Some yoga twists include bringing the hand to the opposite knee—for example, the right hand to left knee—while twisting. This is different: a gentle open twist, practiced mindfully.

- Allow the shoulders to stay relaxed, avoiding hunching.

- Lengthen on the inhale, and twist on the exhale.

MODIFICATION

If it is difficult to come to the floor, you can practice this twist on a chair.

Shoulders, Arms, Wrists, and Hands

Bookmark this page. Each pose and sequence refers to some of the different physical areas and muscle groups shown in this illustration.

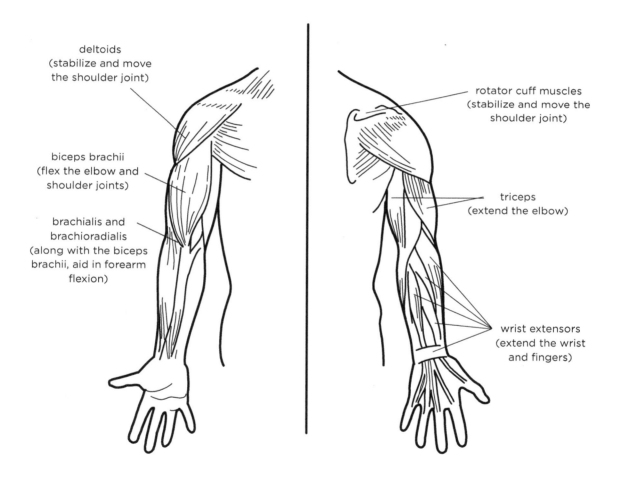

deltoids
(stabilize and move
the shoulder joint)

biceps brachii
(flex the elbow and
shoulder joints)

brachialis and
brachioradialis
(along with the biceps
brachii, aid in forearm
flexion)

rotator cuff muscles
(stabilize and move the
shoulder joint)

triceps
(extend the elbow)

wrist extensors
(extend the wrist
and fingers)

WALL CHEST AND SHOULDER OPENER

PHYSICAL AREAS TARGETED: chest: pectoralis major and minor (see page 68); shoulders and wrists: biceps, wrist extensors

BODY AND MIND AREAS RELIEVED: tight shoulder, tight chest, upper-back rounding, poor posture

This mindful stretch facilitates lengthening and tension release in the chest muscles and along the arm. The only prop needed is a wall, which makes the stretch accessible almost anytime. This opener also facilitates postural awareness and improvement. Practicing this pose reveals how tight our chest and arms can become from extensive sitting or driving and is a wonderful antidote to the accumulation of stressors from a sedentary lifestyle. If you're recovering from chest surgery, be sure to check with your health care provider before doing this pose.

COMMON CONDITIONS ADDRESSED

- Breathing difficulty
- Decreased focus and awareness
- Poor posture

- Shoulder impingement and frozen shoulder recovery
- Tight wrists and forearms

PROPS NEEDED: A WALL

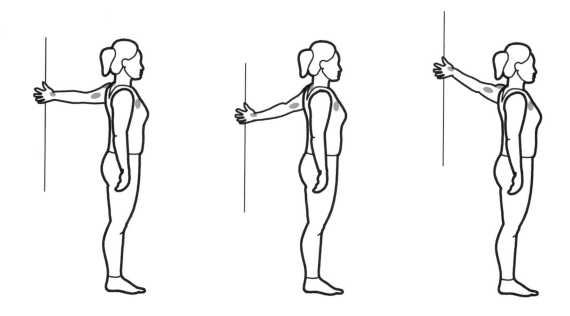

Maintain mountain pose throughout. Arm height can vary.

1. Position yourself in Mountain Pose (see page 33) with the side of your body next to a wall.

2. Bring your hand behind you to the wall, at shoulder height. Turn your fingers away from you.

3. Adjust your hand so you feel lengthening primarily in the chest. You will likely feel the stretch throughout the arm, down to the wrist.

4. After several breaths, pivot your feet and your whole body as one unit 1 or 2 inches away from the wall while keeping your arm and hand in place. This will increase the entire stretch. Modify as necessary so the stretch is not too easy or too difficult.

5. Unwind slowly and stand for a moment before turning to the other side.

6. Repeat with the other arm.

TIPS

- Maintain Mountain Pose (see page 33) throughout every position. Avoid thrusting your ribs or pelvis forward and avoid forward-head posture.

- Pause between sides to breathe and explore the difference between the side that was stretched and the side that wasn't.

MODIFICATION

To stretch your lower and upper pectoral muscles, move your hand slightly lower or higher than shoulder height, and stay for several breaths in the varied positions.

SHOULDER ROTATIONS (FLOSSING)

PHYSICAL AREAS TARGETED: shoulders: rotator cuff muscles, deltoids, rhomboids, biceps, levator scapulae (see page 32); arms: anterior deltoids; chest: pectoralis major (see page 68)

BODY AND MIND AREAS RELIEVED: tightness in the shoulder joints, chest muscles, and chest tissues

This pose maximizes range of motion in the shoulder joints, with the potential of accessing full circumduction. The strap assists in gently facilitating the movement. When you need to reach for an item on a high shelf or grab something from the backseat of a car, you discover the practicality of shoulder rotations for maintaining your shoulder joint mobility. If you take a fall and need to reach for the nearest item to help yourself get back up, you'll be glad you practiced shoulder rotations! The muscles and tissues around the chest also open in this pose for improvement of breath as well as posture.

COMMON CONDITIONS ADDRESSED

- Chest tightness
- General shoulder tightness
- Poor posture
- Shoulder impingement or frozen shoulder
- Wrist tightness

PROPS NEEDED: YOGA STRAP

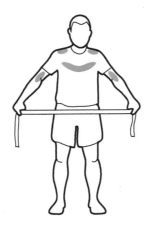 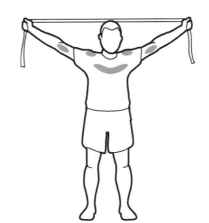 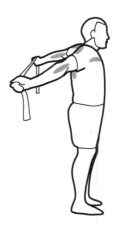

Maintain Mountain Pose the entire time, and go only as far
as current shoulder mobility allows.

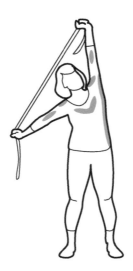

LATERAL STRETCH VARIATION

1. Stand or sit in Mountain Pose.

2. Hold a strap in front of your hips or waist, arms straight and hands wider than shoulder distance apart.

3. Inhale, then lift the strap up, envisioning a semicircle. Do not overly pull or grip the strap. You may not have full mobility in your shoulder joints, depending on your current condition, so go only as far as your range of motion will allow.

4. While keeping your spine in its aligned Mountain Pose position, exhale, then bring the strap over your head and behind you. Slide your hands farther apart if necessary.

5. Smoothly bring the strap back up and over your head to the front of the body.

6. Repeat 5 to 8 times with the breath.

TIPS

- Keep the gaze forward.

- Do not duck your head in order to bring the strap over. Be patient, and go only as far as your range of motion allows.

- Practice coordinating your breath with your movement, and let your jaw remain soft.

MODIFICATION

With the strap over your head, use it to draw the right arm sideways to the left, and then left arm sideways to the right, for lateral stretches of your body.

CACTUS ARMS

PHYSICAL AREAS TARGETED: shoulder (glenohumeral) joints: rotator cuff muscles, especially infraspinatus and teres minor (see page 69); chest muscles: pectoralis (see page 68); back muscles: trapezius (see page 69) and rhomboids (see page 69)

BODY AND MIND AREAS RELIEVED: shoulder tightness, frozen shoulder (with regular practice), tight chest, back tension, lack of concentration, decreased observation, unfocused breathing

Cactus Arms can help you recognize the different range of motion between your shoulders, as well as improve shoulder movement if you practice regularly. This upper-body pose can be done in conjunction with a variety of poses, such as Warrior I (see page 126), Chair Pose (see page 117), and Open Seated Twist (see page 46). Cactus Arms enhances your shoulders' range of motion, opens the chest, and releases back tension. Review this exercise with your health care provider if you are recovering from or are in treatment for a shoulder injury or have a chronic shoulder condition.

COMMON CONDITIONS ADDRESSED

- Arthritis
- Frozen shoulder
- Lack of body awareness and concentration
- Poor posture

PROPS NEEDED: BLANKET (OPTIONAL)

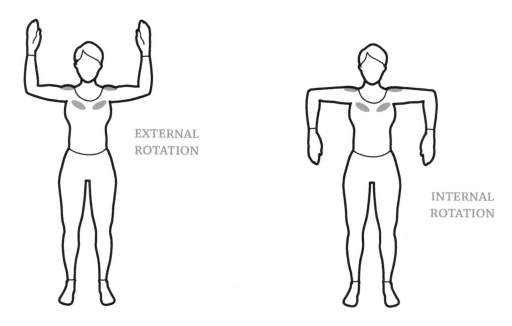

EXTERNAL
ROTATION

INTERNAL
ROTATION

Maintain Mountain Pose the entire time, and go only as far as
current shoulder mobility allows.

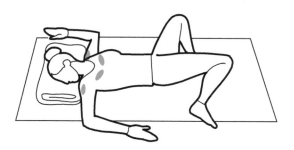

RECLINED ZIGZAG VARIATION: Blanket under hands and
neck; hands may not touch the floor if there are shoulder
restrictions.

1. While seated or standing in Mountain Pose, bring your elbows to shoulder height and slightly behind the shoulder joint. Bend your elbows upward so your palms face forward (external rotation). Slowly draw both elbows away from the body to feel your chest and back opening. Breathe.

2. On your exhale, rotate both shoulder joints (internal rotation) so your palms face behind you and your fingertips point to the floor.

3. Slowly repeat both rotations several times with the breath.

TIPS

- The range of motion will differ between the shoulders based on physical condition and hand dominance, as well as shoulder, back, and chest flexibility.

- Keep the shoulders level and maintain Mountain Pose. Hiking the shoulders up toward the ears or turning the torso to achieve rotation will compromise the flexibility benefits of the pose.

- Coordinate your breath with your movement.

MODIFICATION

For a reclined zigzag variation, lie on your back on your mat with your arms in cactus shape and your knees bent. Turn your head to the left while keeping your chin level as the left arm rotates down and the right arm stays up. Bring your left arm back up. Turn your head right as the right arm rotates down and the left arm stays up. Keep your legs still and keep your scapula connected to the floor even if the hand doesn't touch the floor. The tactile feedback from the mat and floor will give you a sense of progress for increased flexibility.

EAGLE ARMS

PHYSICAL AREAS TARGETED: shoulder muscles: rotator cuff muscles, particularly infraspinatus and teres minor (see page 69), rhomboids; torso muscles: latissimus dorsi (see page 68)

BODY AND MIND AREAS RELIEVED: tight shoulders, tight upper back, stress held in the upper body

Eagle Arms pose and its variations open and lengthen your upper back and shoulders. While you maintain the pose for several steady breaths, the posture provides nuanced insight into the differences between the left and right shoulders. You might notice that your sides have different flexibilities based on which arm is on top. This pose is a wonderful marker of your progress—as your shoulder issues heal over time, you can move from the beginner version to the advanced posture.

COMMON CONDITIONS ADDRESSED

- General upper-body tension
- Shoulder joint impingement, such as frozen shoulder
- Tightness in the wrists
- Upper-back stress and tightness

PROPS NEEDED: BLANKET (OPTIONAL)

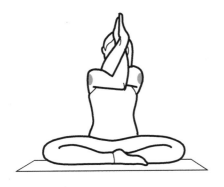
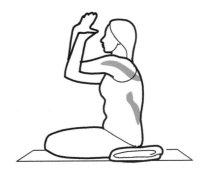

Elbows at shoulder height, forearms away from face.

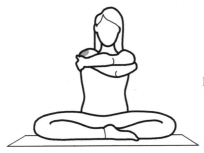
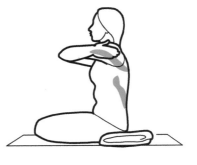

HUG VARIATION

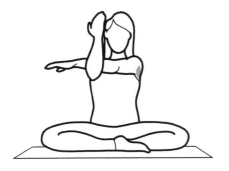

HALF-EAGLE POSE
(variation)

1. Find a comfortable seated position. Bend and bring your elbows and pinkies together with your palms toward your face. Raise both arms to shoulder height. If you can't raise your arms to shoulder height, proceed to the hug variation.

2. Cross the right elbow over the left, maintaining both elbows at shoulder height. Join your palms or join the backs of your hands, depending on the flexibility in your arm joints, your girth, or the size of your chest. Stay relaxed and breathe into the back body for 3 to 5 breaths.

3. Unwind slowly, roll out your shoulders, and stretch your arms out to your sides.

4. Repeat with the left elbow over the right.

TIPS

- Maintain a lengthened spine throughout, keeping your jaw relaxed.

- Enjoy a feeling of broadening between the shoulder blades.

- Draw your elbows away from the face, maintaining them at shoulder height.

MODIFICATIONS

- Give yourself two hugs, alternating the arm that is on top.

- If you have wrist pain or are recovering from shoulder impingement, try the Half-Eagle Pose: Make a hook at about a 90-degree angle with your elbow. Place the opposite arm on the hook. Breathe into the stretch, particularly at the scapula and side body, and play with movement.

WRIST AND FOREARM STRETCH

PHYSICAL AREAS TARGETED: forearm flexors and extensors of the wrists and hands

BODY AND MIND AREAS RELIEVED: tightness in the wrists and forearms

Wrist soreness is a common by-product of repetitive motion. Activities such as knitting, texting, typing, and practicing a musical instrument can trigger over-use soreness and imbalances in the wrist. This pose uses the yin style and helps strengthen and lengthen your wrists. It will help protect this joint or support recovery from a previous injury. If you have arthritis pain, make sure you use gentle movements. This sequence is designed to maintain and increase the health of the tissues around the wrists and forearms. If this stretch exacerbates pain from any preexisting conditions, see a health care provider or decrease the range of motion of the movements. If you're recovering from a wrist sprain or a fracture, make sure you consult with a medical professional before doing this pose.

COMMON CONDITIONS ADDRESSED

- Arthritis
- Carpal tunnel
- Recovery from a sprain or fracture
- Soreness from typing and texting
- Wrist pain from feeding a baby
- Wrist tendinitis

PROPS NEEDED: TABLE (OPTIONAL)

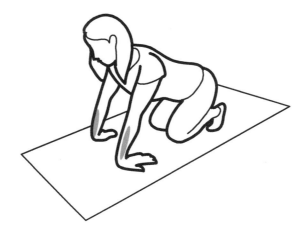

Move hips slowly toward feet until you feel a stretch in the wrists and forearms.

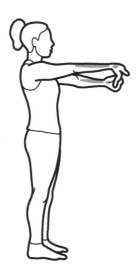

STANDING VARIATION

1. Warm up your wrists by making easy circle motions. You can keep your fingers open or closed. You can move both wrists at once or one at a time. Rotate them clockwise and counterclockwise.

2. Come to your hands and knees (Table Pose) on a mat. Align your wrists under your shoulders and your knees under your hip joints. Rotate your fingertips outward. Sway your body left and right as you feel lengthening in the forearms and wrists.

3. Keep your palms down and turn the hands so your fingertips are facing your knees. Gently move your body slightly away from your fingertips, keeping the heels of your hands on the floor until you feel a stretching or lengthening sensation. Hold for up to a minute and breathe.

4. Repeat the wrist circles.

TIPS

- If it is difficult or impractical to come to the floor, perform this exercise at a table. Sit or stand in front of a table and practice the same series with your palms on the table instead of the floor.

- Practice this yin stretch throughout the day.

MODIFICATION

Start with Mountain Pose (see page 33). Stretch your right arm out in front of you, palm facing up. Stretch your right wrist with the left hand by gently pulling the fingers toward you. Repeat with your left arm.

SUPPORTED BACKBEND

PHYSICAL AREAS TARGETED: chest and torso: pectoralis major and minor, serratus anterior (see page 68); mid back: thoracic spine; shoulders: deltoids

BODY AND MIND AREAS RELIEVED: tightness in the chest, shoulders, upper back and neck

This restorative and yin pose works with gravity to counteract tension in the chest, shoulders, and mid back. As you remain in the pose, restriction in the tissues slowly unwinds and stickiness around the shoulders and chest is relieved, allowing for better breath and posture. The joy of this pose also includes meditative focus and a sense of peaceful release of all that we carry in our muscles and our minds.

COMMON CONDITIONS ADDRESSED

- Decreased relaxation response
- Postural dysfunction
- Shallow breathing
- Shoulder impingement and frozen shoulder
- Some forms of asthma
- Stress

PROPS NEEDED: BLANKET(S), BLOCK (OPTIONAL), CLOTH (OPTIONAL)

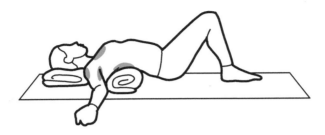

Optional blanket under the head and neck.

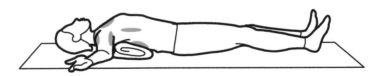

The knees can be bent or straight.

1. Place a rolled towel or blanket across your mat.

2. Lie down so your mid back is on the support. The lower part of your shoulder blades may also be supported.

3. Adjust so your shoulders are on the floor and your armpits are not on the support.

4. Bring your arms to a T shape and position them above the support.

5. Your leg positions can vary—you can place your feet on the floor with your knees bent or keep your legs straight.

6. Breathe slowly and remain in this shape for 2 to 5 minutes.

7. Come out of the pose slowly and consciously by bending your knees, rolling to one side, and removing the prop. Once the prop is out of the way, lie on your back with your knees bent or pulled to your chest for several breaths.

8. Roll to your side and press up with your arm strength.

TIP

The prop height will vary. You can stack up to three blankets depending on your current back, chest, and shoulder mobility and flexibility.

MODIFICATIONS

- Place a blanket or block under your head and neck.

- Place a cloth over your eyes for further relaxation.

Chest, Torso, and Back

Bookmark this page! Each pose and sequence refers to the different physical areas and muscle groups shown in this illustration.

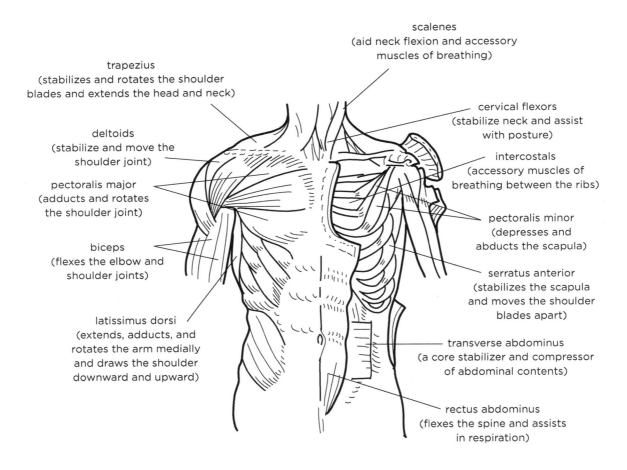

scalenes
(aid neck flexion and accessory muscles of breathing)

trapezius
(stabilizes and rotates the shoulder blades and extends the head and neck)

cervical flexors
(stabilize neck and assist with posture)

deltoids
(stabilize and move the shoulder joint)

intercostals
(accessory muscles of breathing between the ribs)

pectoralis major
(adducts and rotates the shoulder joint)

pectoralis minor
(depresses and abducts the scapula)

biceps
(flexes the elbow and shoulder joints)

serratus anterior
(stabilizes the scapula and moves the shoulder blades apart)

latissimus dorsi
(extends, adducts, and rotates the arm medially and draws the shoulder downward and upward)

transverse abdominus
(a core stabilizer and compressor of abdominal contents)

rectus abdominus
(flexes the spine and assists in respiration)

FRONT

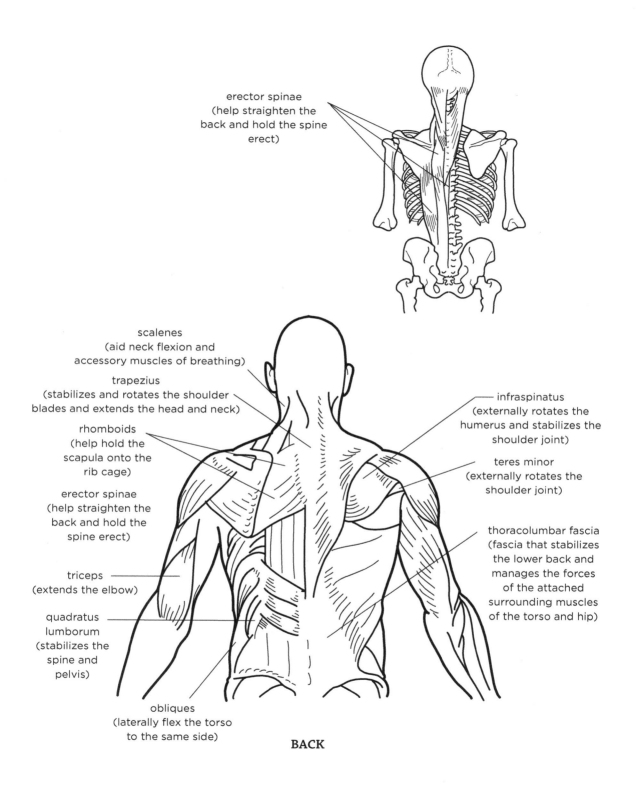

erector spinae
(help straighten the
back and hold the spine
erect)

scalenes
(aid neck flexion and
accessory muscles of breathing)

trapezius
(stabilizes and rotates the shoulder
blades and extends the head and neck)

rhomboids
(help hold the
scapula onto the
rib cage)

erector spinae
(help straighten the
back and hold the
spine erect)

triceps
(extends the elbow)

quadratus
lumborum
(stabilizes the
spine and
pelvis)

obliques
(laterally flex the torso
to the same side)

infraspinatus
(externally rotates the
humerus and stabilizes the
shoulder joint)

teres minor
(externally rotates the
shoulder joint)

thoracolumbar fascia
(fascia that stabilizes
the lower back and
manages the forces
of the attached
surrounding muscles
of the torso and hip)

BACK

DOWNWARD-FACING DOG

PHYSICAL AREAS TARGETED: arms and shoulders: triceps, deltoids, rhomboids, trapezius, infraspinatus, and teres minor; spine: erector spinae, latissimus dorsi; legs: hamstrings, gastrocnemius (see page 154)

BODY AND MIND AREAS RELIEVED: tight shoulder joints; restricted diaphragm; stiff spine, legs, and arms; anxiety and worry

Downward-Facing Dog strengthens the muscles and bones while stretching the entire body. It is a partial inversion that helps bring circulation to the upper body, simultaneously benefiting your body, mind, and breath. You can increase flexibility to your hamstrings, feet, and toes, and stimulate the bones of your spine, wrists, and pelvis. You can see the world from an entirely different point of view in this classic yoga pose.

COMMON CONDITIONS ADDRESSED

- Back pain
- Menopause symptoms
- Osteoporosis
- Pelvic pain

- Tightness in the hamstrings and calves
- Weakness in the arms

PROPS NEEDED: WALL OR CHAIR (OPTIONAL)

1. Come to your hands and knees (Table Pose) on a mat. Align the wrists under the

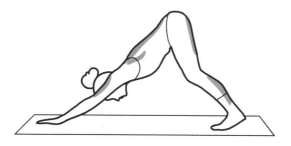

Bend the knees slightly to lengthen the
spine—the heels may not come to the floor.

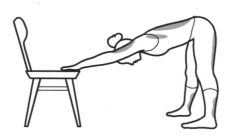

CHAIR VARIATION: Practice chair dog if your wrists
are tender and you don't want to go to the floor.

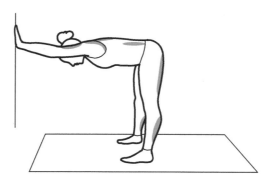

WALL VARIATION: Modification for glaucoma, high
blood pressure, vertigo, later stages of pregnancy.

shoulders and the knees under the hip joints.

2. Move your wrists slightly in front of your shoulders, and make sure your wrist creases are parallel to the front of the mat. Press into the pads of all 10 fingers to distribute the weight evenly in your hands.

3. Press the floor away from you strongly while moving your hips up and back.

4. Keep your knees slightly bent, legs hip distance apart, and toes forward.

5. Maintain the natural curve of the spine and avoid rounding at the lumbar spine. Your heels may not touch the floor, and your knees can stay slightly bent so you can find space in your spine.

6. Feel your shoulder blades move apart and away from your ears.

7. Press your hands into the mat as though you're making an imprint in the sand.

8. Breathe, be strong, be playful. Walk the dog by bending one knee and then the other. Build up to holding this pose for up to 10 breaths.

9. To move out of the pose, slowly let your knees come to the floor and then take a Child's Pose by bringing the big toes together, knees apart. Stack your hands under your forehead, draw your hips back toward your heels, and rest.

TIP

Don't allow the weight of your head to draw your chin to your chest.

MODIFICATIONS

- Practice the chair dog variation if you have wrist issues, untreated high blood pressure, or chronic vertigo. Stand in front of a stable chair and place your hands on the back or seat, shoulder distance apart. Walk back from the chair until your spine is lengthened, feet hip distance apart or wider. Bend your knees and slide your hips back if your back is rounding. To come out of the pose, walk back in toward the chair and move into Mountain Pose.

- Practice the wall dog variation if you have glaucoma, untreated high blood pressure, or chronic vertigo. Stand in front of a wall and place your hands on it, shoulder distance apart and slightly above your shoulders. Walk back from the wall until your spine is lengthened, feet hip distance apart or wider. Bend your knees and slide your hips back if your back is rounding. To come out of this pose, walk in toward the wall.

WIDE-LEG HALF FORWARD BEND

PHYSICAL AREAS TARGETED: back: erector spinae muscles; hips: gluteus maximus, pelvic floor (see page 110); legs: hamstrings, gastrocnemius (see page 154)

BODY AND MIND AREAS RELIEVED: tight hamstrings, sore back, poor posture, restricted breathing

Wide-Leg Half Forward Bend is a symmetrical pose that brings flexibility and stability to the back of the body. It is safe for almost everyone, including pregnant women, as the position avoids rounding out and pressuring the lumbar spine. Since the head does not drop below the heart, the shape can also be safe for those with glaucoma. If the spine does round, or if you have disc issues or severe osteoporosis, you can practice this pose at a table or a kitchen counter. Your pelvic floor, hamstrings, and calf muscles will lengthen and release tension.

COMMON CONDITIONS ADDRESSED

- Back pain

- Hypertonic pelvic floor

- Stress

- Tight legs

- Vertigo (has the benefits of a forward fold without bringing the head lower than the heart in the table version)

- Weak core

PROPS NEEDED: BLOCK(S), TABLE OR WALL (OPTIONAL)

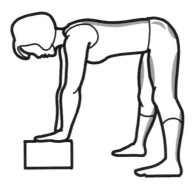

Keep your wrists under your shoulders, heels
wider than your hips, with your toes forward.

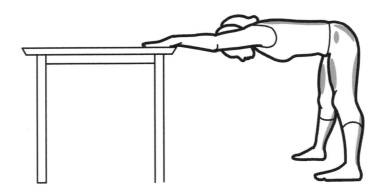

TABLE VARIATION: Support your
wrists on a table, with your toes forward.

1. Place a block or two in front of your feet.

2. Stand with your legs wider than hip distance apart, toes forward, and hands on your pelvis.

3. Spread your weight evenly on the inner and outer arches of your feet.

4. Inhale deeply, all the way down your spine and into the pelvis.

5. On your exhale, bend forward from the hip joints. Make sure you avoid rounding your back.

6. Bring your fingertips or hands to the block (or blocks) and keep your spine parallel to the floor.

7. Slide your shoulders away from your ears while gently lengthening your chest forward. Bring slightly more weight to your heels.

8. Keep your head and neck in line with your entire spine. Inhale down your spine and into the pelvic floor. On your exhale, feel your belly, ribs, and back contract. Practice 360-degree breathing (see page 13) for several breaths.

9. To come out of the pose, walk your feet toward the midline of the body and bring your hands to your hips. On an exhale, bring your torso upright to standing.

10. Take Mountain Pose for a few breaths and feel the benefits of the pose.

TIP

Sense your chest moving forward and your hips moving back so your spine is parallel to the floor.

MODIFICATIONS

- If you have glaucoma or vertigo, or if it is difficult to reach a stack of two blocks, practice the pose at a table, counter, or wall. Place your hands on the table, wrists supported. Walk back until you feel full length in your spine and then bring your feet wider than hip distance apart. Continue the posture with steps 7 through 10.

- Once you are in the pose, you may be able to widen your stance. When doing so, keep pressing into the inner and outer arches of the feet, feeling the inner thighs engage.

SUNBIRD POSE

PHYSICAL AREAS TARGETED: back: erector spinae; core: rectus abdominus, obliques, transverse abdominus; lower body: gluteals, hamstrings, iliopsoas (see page 110)

BODY AND MIND AREAS RELIEVED: back pain, poor posture, weak core, scattered mind

Sunbird Pose is sometimes called Bird Dog Pose. This dynamic pose is a simple and effective core stabilizer and strengthener that can also relieve back pain and enhance balance. Shoulder mobility, concentration, and focus are improved. Spinal stability and alignment are enhanced. This pose is safe for pregnant women or individuals with osteoporosis.

COMMON CONDITIONS ADDRESSED

- Back pain
- Balance difficulties
- Instability in daily life
- Lack of breathing coordination and focus
- Unhealthy postural alignment
- Unstable spine

PROPS NEEDED: BLANKET (OPTIONAL), CHAIR (OPTIONAL)

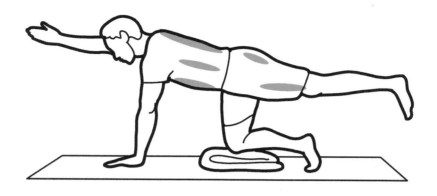

Keep your hips level.

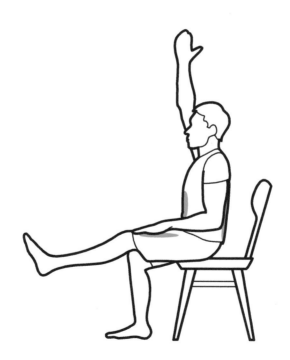

CHAIR VARIATION: Keep your spine lengthened.

1. Come to your hands and knees (Table Pose) on a mat. Align your wrists under your shoulders and knees under your hip joints. Remember to press into the pads of all 10 fingers to take pressure off your wrists.

2. Slowly bring your left leg off the mat and straighten the knee. The leg should be level or slightly lower than the hip, not higher. Breathe consciously.

3. Bring your right arm off the floor with the palm facing the midline of the body. Engage your core muscles to stabilize. Lengthen your fingertips forward and your leg back.

4. After several breaths, return to Table Pose and repeat on the other side.

5. Work toward 5 repetitions on each side.

TIPS

- Keep your neck and head even with the rest of your spine, as though you are standing in Mountain Pose. Your gaze can be slightly down or out in front of you.

- Avoid shifting your hips or shoulders to one side or the other. Imagine there is a cup of tea on your sacrum that you don't want to spill. Place a yoga block there to remind yourself to keep your hips level.

- Don't let the front body sag toward the floor.

MODIFICATIONS

- Place a double-folded blanket under your knees for extra support.

- If it is too difficult to raise both your arm and leg together, work in increments. For example, start with raising the leg only and keeping both hands on the floor.

- If you are unable to come to the floor, practice the chair modification. Sit up straight toward the front of the chair, feet flat on the ground and hip distance apart. Inhale, raise your left arm to shoulder height or higher, and lift your right leg off the floor. Exhale and lower the arm and leg, then raise the right arm and left leg, continuing at a moderate pace, working toward 5 repetitions on each side.

YOGA HEEL DROPS

PHYSICAL AREAS TARGETED: core: rectus abdominus, transverse abdominus; hip flexor: iliopsoas (see page 110)

BODY AND MIND AREAS RELIEVED: lower-back pain, abdominal muscle weakness

A strong functioning core is important for maintaining good posture, sustaining back health, and going about daily activities. You can perform Yoga Heel Drops safely regardless of your strength level; as you gain strength, progress to the straight-leg variation. Keep your head on the floor throughout the pose to avoid the neck stress that many people experience while doing traditional abdominal crunches.

COMMON CONDITIONS ADDRESSED

- Back strain
- Balance difficulties
- Core weakness
- Diminished strength after pregnancy
- Pelvic imbalances
- Poor posture
- Reduced body stability

PROPS NEEDED: FOLDED BLANKET (OPTIONAL)

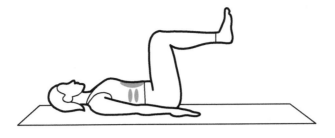

Start with your knees over your hips.

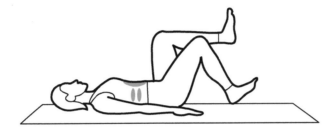

Move your heel out several inches from the hip
when your heel touches the floor.

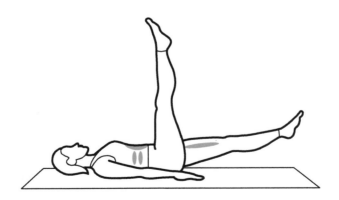

CHALLENGING STRAIGHT-LEG VARIATION:
Keep the ribs from jutting toward the ceiling.

1. Lie on your back with both knees bent, feet on the floor. Keep your arms by your sides.

2. Lift both feet off the floor, keeping your bent knees aligned over your hips.

3. Alternate touching one heel at a time to the floor approximately 6 inches away from the hips. Keep the leg in the same bent-knee shape the entire time.

4. While performing this exercise, sense that your bottom ribs are connected to the floor and feel that your abdominal muscles are engaged. If you find your ribs are jutting toward the ceiling and you feel your lower back arching, don't lower your heel all the way to the floor. Once you build up more strength, you can inch your heel closer to the floor.

5. Start with 5 repetitions on each leg, increasing the repetitions until you can practice for approximately 60 seconds.

TIPS

- Imagine there's space to place a grape under your lumbar spine so you maintain the natural curve of your lower back.

- Place a blanket under your head and neck for comfort, or if your chin is straining toward the ceiling.

MODIFICATION

To make this exercise more challenging, straighten your legs more. Keep your mind focused on your core. Make sure your ribs aren't jutting toward the ceiling and your back isn't arched.

RECLINED SPINAL TWIST

PHYSICAL AREAS TARGETED: bones of the spine; core muscles, particularly the obliques and transverse abdominus; chest muscles: pectoralis (see page 68); neck muscles: scalenes (see page 32)

BODY AND MIND AREAS RELIEVED: back pain, chest tightness, shoulder tightness, restricted breathing

You can practice this versatile reclined twist as a yin or restorative passive tissue release, or as a core-strengthening pose and tension reliever. In either version, the skin of the belly, the internal organs, and the spine muscles and bones are awakened and stimulated. Reclined Spinal Twist helps you maintain and nurture the practical ability to gently rotate the spine if you need to reach behind you, or if you have been sedentary at work, in daily life, or from travel. This is a good counterpose to backbends, such as Sphinx Pose (see page 85).

COMMON CONDITIONS ADDRESSED

- Back pain
- Constricted breathing
- Core weakness

- Shoulder and chest tightness
- Stress

PROPS NEEDED: BLANKET (OPTIONAL)

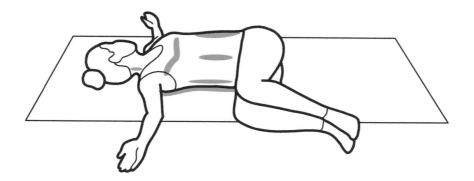

Keep your spine long, knees even with the hips.

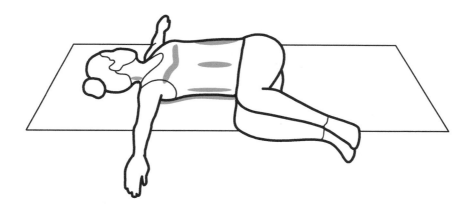

STRENGTHENING VARIATION: Keep your palms
down and hover the legs above the floor for 1 to 3
breaths.

1. Lie on the floor. Bend both knees and lift both feet off the floor. Keep your legs, knees, and ankles together (as much as your bone and muscle structure allow), as though your legs were one unit.

2. Bring your arms to either a T shape (palms up) or Cactus Arms (see page 56). Bring both legs together to rest on the right side of the body.

3. Turn your face to the ceiling. If you are safely able, turn your face slightly to the right to enhance the stretch in the neck muscles and cervical spine.

4. Feel length and space in the waist, lower back, belly, and chest.

5. Rest in this shape for 5 breaths, or for a deeper yin-style practice, hold for 2 to 4 minutes.

6. Maintain easy breathing throughout.

7. To come out of this pose, use gentle core strength to bring your legs up. Rest with your feet on the ground and compare the effects of the pose on both sides of the body.

8. Repeat on the other side, bringing your legs to the right and your face to the left.

TIPS

- To maintain length in the spine, keep the knees level with the hip joints. This prevents your back from rounding and your body from coiling into a fetal position.

- Place a folded blanket under the knees and legs if you have trouble resting them on the floor without the opposite shoulder joint lifting too much.

MODIFICATION

To practice as a core-strengthening pose, repeat steps 1 through 4. Face your palms downward instead of up, and instead of resting your legs on the floor, use your core strength to hover the legs a few inches off the floor, holding for up to 3 breaths. Feel the obliques engage. After 3 breaths, use your core strength to bring your legs to the opposite side to hover. Repeat 4 to 8 times on each side.

SPHINX POSE

PHYSICAL AREAS TARGETED: spine: erector spinae; chest: pectoralis muscles and tissues around the lungs; arms: biceps and triceps

BODY AND MIND AREAS RELIEVED: tight back muscles, diminished breath capacity

Sphinx is a mild backbend you can practice in yin style (held for 2 to 5 minutes) or in yang style for a few conscious breaths, resting and then repeating. The easeful spinal extension with the support of the floor safely stimulates the bones of the back and opens the chest and lungs to increase breathing capacity. If you have spinal disc conditions or other issues, check with your health care provider to make sure spinal extension movements (backbends) are okay for you.

COMMON CONDITIONS ADDRESSED

- Back muscle weakness
- Back pain
- Decreased breath awareness and capacity
- Osteoporosis
- Poor posture
- Tension and stress

PROPS NEEDED: MAT (OPTIONAL), BLANKET (OPTIONAL), BLOCK (OPTIONAL), WALL (OPTIONAL)

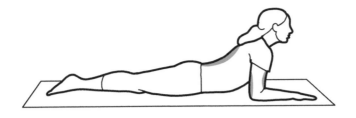

Relax your shoulders away from your ears.

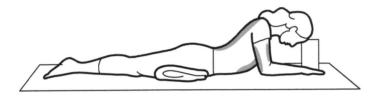

YIN-STYLE VARIATION: Optional blanket under the hips.

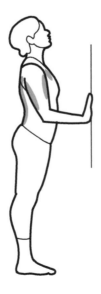

WALL VARIATION: Lengthen the spine.

1. Lie on your belly and bring your legs hip distance apart.

2. Place the elbows under the shoulders, with your forearms parallel to each other.

3. Ensure your pubic bone is in gentle contact with the floor, and wiggle your hips left and right to sense symmetry. Avoid gripping the gluteal muscles.

4. Rest on the floor, stacking your hands under your forehead. Relax your face and jaw. Feel the rise and fall of several breaths.

5. Practice a counterpose, such as Reclined Spinal Twist (see page 82).

TIPS

- Place a mat or other padding under your elbows and hips for comfort.

- Keep your chest open and avoid gripping or overly shrugging in the shoulder joints.

- Imagine a sense of spaciousness along the vertebrae.

MODIFICATIONS

- If you'd like to practice in the yin style (holding the pose for 2 to 5 minutes), try placing a block under your forehead to avoid neck strain.

- Feel free to adjust your legs to be slightly wider or narrower than hip distance if that feels most comfortable for your lower back and pelvis.

- If you can't lie on your belly, try the wall variation. Stand in Mountain Pose 6 to 8 inches from a wall and place your hands approximately chest high on the wall. Firmly press your hands into the wall and feel your spine extend in and up without letting your head drop back. Breathe in this posture for up to 5 breaths.

SUPPORTED BRIDGE ON BLOCK

PHYSICAL AREAS TARGETED: upper body: pectoralis, deltoids, biceps; lower body: quadriceps (see page 133), psoas (see page 110)

BODY AND MIND AREAS RELIEVED: tight chest, tight hip flexors, overall muscle tension accumulated from stress

Supported Bridge on Block allows the pull of gravity to relieve tightness in the front of the body. Because your head is lower than your heart in this position, your parasympathetic nervous system is engaged for relaxation enhancement. Your posture will improve as chest and shoulder tension unravels in this gently supported backbend. If you have an abdominal hernia, a recent anterior hip replacement, or a herniated disc, check with your health care provider before doing this pose.

COMMON CONDITIONS ADDRESSED

- Head-forward posture
- Reduced breathing capacity
- Sacroiliac joint pain

- Stress
- Tight chest

PROPS NEEDED: BLOCK (OR FIRM FOLDED BLANKETS)

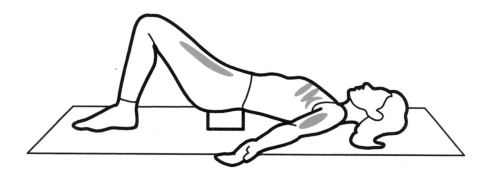

Block under sacrum. Optional to
bring block to a higher height.

1. Lie on the mat with your knees bent.

2. Press into your feet and lift your hips. Slide the block at its lowest height directly underneath your sacrum. Adjust the block with your hands until it feels balanced. Be sure the block is underneath the sacrum, not the lower spine.

3. Bring your heels underneath or slightly in front of your knees, depending on the comfort level of your hip flexors.

4. Roll your shoulders slightly underneath your chest and face your palms up. Relax your forehead, jaw, and the skin of your face.

5. Rest in the pose for 4 to 10 minutes.

6. To come out of the pose, press into your feet, lift your hips, and remove the block. Pause and breathe.

TIPS

- Counterposes include Open Seated Twist (see page 46) or Reclined Spinal Twist (see page 82).

- In this pose, as in all restorative or yin postures, we practice allowing yourself to be rather than do. Enjoy this meditative aspect of the pose.

- If you don't have a block, or if a block feels too hard, fold 1 or 2 firm blankets and place them under your hips.

- Consider setting a timer to ensure you are in the pose long enough for benefits to accrue.

MODIFICATION

For a deeper stretch, after a few moments reach underneath and rest the block on a medium height side to make it higher. For the deepest stretch, stand the block on the highest level.

Upper-Body Sequences

POSTURE FOCUS

PHYSICAL AREAS TARGETED

This sequence relieves tightness in the chest and shoulders that results from poor postural habits and stress. The series lengthens the muscles and tissues around the neck, shoulders, and back that become habitually bound from less-than-optimal daily routines. Notice your poised and improved stance once you get to Mountain Pose. The spinal strength, awareness, and length gained from Sphinx Pose and the shoulder and hip release from the Cactus Arms reclined zigzag variation support your Mountain Pose. When you find room in the chest and avoid slumping, you can breathe freely and calmly.

Head and Neck Muscles (see page 32)
- levator scapulae
- semispinalis capitis
- sternocleidomastoid

Shoulder, Arm, Wrist, and Hand Muscles (see page 49)
- biceps
- rotator cuff muscles

Chest, Torso, and Back (see pages 68-69)
- cervical flexors
- erector spinae
- pectoralis muscles
- rhomboids
- trapezius

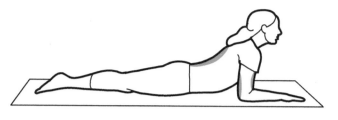

1. SPHINX POSE

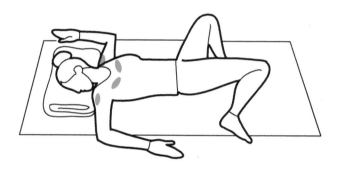

2. CACTUS ARMS
reclined zigzag variation

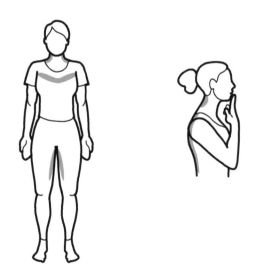

3. MOUNTAIN POSE

1. Begin lying on your belly with your legs hip distance apart. Practice Sphinx Pose (see page 85) for several breaths or yin-style Sphinx Pose for a minimum of 2 minutes. Then rest on your belly with your hands stacked under your forehead for several breaths.

2. For Cactus Arms with reclined zigzag variation, come to your back, then bring your feet hip distance apart and your arms into Cactus Arms (see page 56). Rotate arms and legs in opposite rotations on both sides for several breaths. Then rest on your back with your knees bent, or draw your knees to your chest.

3. Make your way to standing. Practice Mountain Pose (see page 33) and add the chin-tuck action.

TIP

Practice supportive affirmations, such as "I move through life with poise" or "I am a balance of strength and ease."

MODIFICATION

If coming to the floor is unavailable, practice standing Cactus Arms, Sphinx Pose wall variation, and seated Mountain Pose.

STRENGTH FOCUS

PHYSICAL AREAS TARGETED

A strong core supports our everyday movements such as rising from a chair, lifting a child or a bag of groceries, doing laundry, or washing dishes. Our core is critical for balance and posture, and core strength prevents back pain. This sequence provides back stabilization and overall core endurance and strength with Yoga Heel Drops and Sunbird Pose. Moving to Downward-Facing Dog, you will simultaneously lengthen and release the spine and build strength in your arms (including your wrists), hips, and legs.

Shoulder, Arm, Wrist, and Hand Muscles (see page 49)

- deltoids
- rotator cuff
- triceps

Chest, Torso, and Back Muscles (see pages 68–69)

- erector spinae
- latissimus dorsi
- obliques
- rectus abdominus
- rhomboids
- trapezius
- traverse abdominus

Hip, Gluteal, and Pelvic Muscles (see page 110)

- gluteal muscles
- iliopsoas

Thigh and Knee Muscles (see page 133)

- hamstrings

Calves, Ankles, and Feet (see page 154)

- gastrocnemius

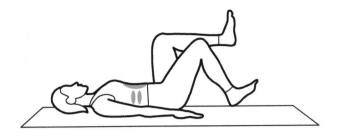

1. YOGA HEEL DROPS POSE

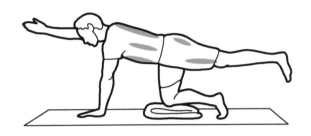

2. SUNBIRD POSE

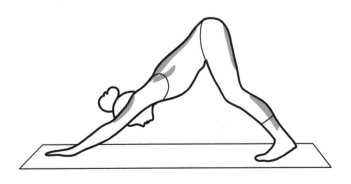

3. DOWNWARD-FACING DOG POSE

1. Lie on your back with both knees bent. Place a blanket under your head and neck. Practice Yoga Heel Drops (see page 79) for 5 or more repetitions on each leg. Take a nice full-body stretch or hug your knees to your chest.

2. Moving to all fours on your mat, place the blanket under your knees, if needed. Practice Sunbird Pose (see page 76) for up to 5 or more repetitions on each side. Rest and rotate your wrists or move directly into the next pose.

3. From all fours, place your wrists slightly in front of your shoulder joints and press the floor away as your hips move toward the sky in Downward-Facing Dog (see page 70) for 5 to 10 breaths.

4. From Downward-Facing Dog, walk your hands toward your feet and your feet toward hands. Hinge up to standing to Mountain Pose for several breaths. Feel the strength and empowerment stimulated by this sequence.

TIPS

- Beware of holding tension in your jaw while practicing this strengthening sequence.

- Practice positive affirmations, such as "Yoga self-care gives me strength" or "My muscles, my breath, and my mind become stronger as I practice."

- If you are in recovery from an illness and rebuilding strength, rest a bit longer between poses, take fewer repetitions, or practice the modification.

MODIFICATION

If you are unable to come to the floor for these poses, try seated Sunbird Pose in lieu of Yoga Heel Drops, and wall or chair Downward-Facing Dog.

FLEXIBILITY FOCUS

PHYSICAL AREAS TARGETED

If you've been sedentary or inactive because of work, an illness, travel, or even binge-watching a streaming series, your body and mind will appreciate this upper-body flexibility sequence. A stiff neck, a tight back and hips, and tense shoulders are signs that it is time to move. After you release the neck and shoulders, your entire spine will extend and flex so you can free stiff muscles and tissues and hydrate them with movement. This sequence ends with a gentle spinal twist that opens your back body and unravels any remaining stiffness as the chest opens and receives the breath.

Head and Neck Muscles (see page 32)

- levator scapulae
- scalenes
- splenius capitis, splenius cervicis
- sternocleidomastoid

Chest, Torso, and Back Muscles (see pages 68–69)

- erector spinae
- obliques
- pectoralis
- transverse abdominus
- trapezius, upper back, and posterior neck

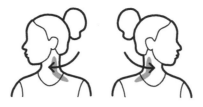

1. NECK ROTATIONS

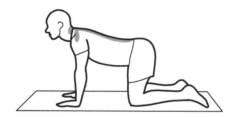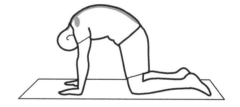

2. CAT/COW

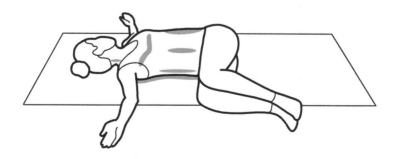

3. RECLINED SPINAL TWIST

1. Start in any seated position. Breathe consciously and mindfully, observing whether there is any tension in your shoulders, neck, or jaw. Practice Neck Rotations with Optional Manual Traction (see page 37). When you have completed the series, observe the changes in your physical and mental stress levels.

2. Come to hands and knees on the mat and practice Cat/Cow with Neck-Focused Turtle (see page 40). Repeat as many times as you wish, then lie down on your back with bent knees.

3. Practice Reclined Spinal Twist (see page 82) on both sides for several breaths or yin style for 2 to 4 minutes on each side. Rest with your knees bent, hands on your belly. Feel your breath.

TIP

Practice the following affirmations: "My spine deserves this practice" and "My healing practice is dissolving tension and stress."

MODIFICATION

You can practice the entire sequence in a chair: Neck Rotations with Optional Manual Traction, Cat/Cow chair variation, and Open Seated Twist chair variation.

A LITTLE BIT OF EVERYTHING

PHYSICAL AREAS TARGETED

Part of the fun of this sequence is working with yoga props and pose variations that provide access to movements that might otherwise be physically difficult. The blocks or table in Wide-Leg Half Forward Bend allows us to feel spacious in the spine, fold forward, and employ our core strength without rounding the back. The Open Seated Twist is a very gentle and safe way to stimulate the spine and internal organs without putting undue pressure on the vertebrae.

Head and Neck Muscles (see page 32)
- levator scapulae
- scalenes
- sternocleidomastoid

Shoulder, Arm, Wrist, and Hand Muscles (see page 49)
- biceps
- deltoids
- rotator cuff muscles

Chest, Torso, and Back Muscles (see pages 68–69)
- erector spinae
- obliques
- pectoralis muscles
- rhomboids

Hip, Gluteal, and Pelvic Muscles (see page 110)
- gluteal muscles
- pelvic floor

Thigh and Knee Muscles (see page 133)
- hamstrings

Calf, Ankle, and Foot Muscles (see page 154)
- gastrocnemius

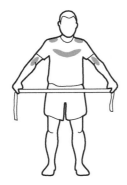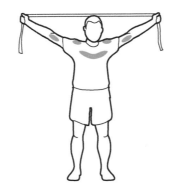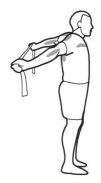

1. SHOULDER ROTATIONS

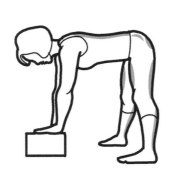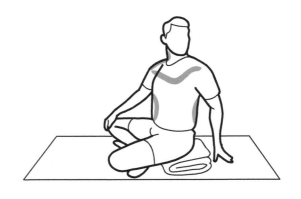

2. WIDE-LEG HALF FORWARD BEND   3. OPEN SEATED TWIST

1. With a yoga strap or tie while standing in Mountain Pose (see page 33), practice Shoulder Rotations (see page 53) 5 to 8 times with the breath. Returning to Mountain Pose, feel the surge of vitality from opening the shoulders and chest.

2. You can practice Wide-Leg Half Forward Bend with yoga blocks or at a table. With your hands on your hips and legs wide apart, inhale and hinge at the hip into the pose (see page 73). Inhabit the pose for several breaths. Mindfully exit the pose.

3. Make your way to the floor and practice Open Seated Twist (see page 46) for several breaths on each side. Make sure to sit on a blanket if your spine is rounding. Stay seated and spend a few minutes in your choice of meditation.

TIPS

- Have your strap, blanket, and blocks ready prior to practicing this sequence.

- Practice the following affirmations: "My body and mind are on a healing path" and "I trust my practice to support my healing."

MODIFICATION

From seated Mountain Pose, practice seated Shoulder Rotations and Open Seated Twist in a chair. Include Wide-Leg Half Forward Bend if you are able to stand.

UNWIND AND DE-STRESS

PHYSICAL AREAS TARGETED

Your upper and mid back, and then the entire spine and hip flexors, will benefit from letting go of physical stress and mental tension in this upper-body-focused yin/restorative sequence. Allow gravity to undo issues in your tissues (tight muscles, stiff joints, and sticky fascia) that are the result of repetitive postural habits and mental anxiety. We have discussed the stress-reducing effects of yoga on all layers of our being (koshas). This series employs easy yogic breathing while practicing.

Head and Neck Muscles (see page 32)
- splenius capitis, splenius cervicis
- trapezius
- upper back and posterior neck

Shoulder, Arm, Wrist, and Hand Muscles (see page 49)
- deltoids
- rhomboids

Chest, Torso, and Back Muscles (see pages 68–69)
- pectoralis muscles
- rotator cuff muscles
- serratus anterior

Hip, Gluteal, and Pelvic Muscles (see page 110)
- hip flexors: iliopsoas and rectus femoris

Thigh and Knee Muscles (see page 133)
- quadriceps

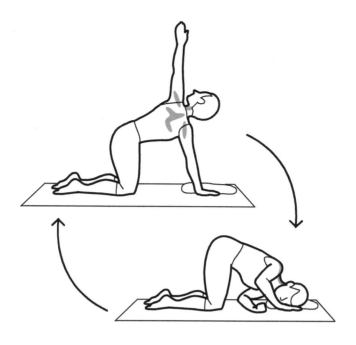

1. THREAD THE NEEDLE

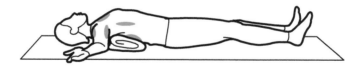

2. SUPPORTED BACKBEND

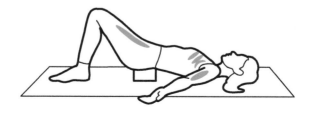

3. SUPPORTED BRIDGE ON BLOCK

1. Come to your hands and knees (Table Pose) on a mat. Align your wrists under your shoulders and your knees under your hip joints. Practice Thread the Needle (see page 43), relaxing for 5 or 6 breaths on each side. When you come out of the pose, roll your shoulders forward and backward a few times and notice the tension release.

2. Place your rolled blanket or towel across your mat and lie down on top of it so your mid back is supported. Enjoy Supported Backbend (see page 65) for 2 to 5 minutes. To come out, remove the blanket and relax on your back with your knees bent for several breaths.

3. Press into your feet, lift your hips, and place your block directly beneath your hips under the sacrum (not the lower back). Rest in Supported Bridge on Block (see page 88) for 4 to 10 minutes.

TIPS

- Make sure you have 1 or 2 blankets and a block nearby before beginning the practice.

- A timer or stopwatch (check your phone for these tools, but make sure the ringer is off!) is handy when practicing yin and restorative poses. Set your timer for each pose, relax, and let the postures do their magic.

- Create the external conditions for letting go and relaxing by ensuring your space is quiet, warm, lit softly, or dark.

- Feel free to play unobtrusive relaxing instrumental music when you are first practicing. Over time, you may not need or want it.

- To calm the mind and offer self-support, repeat to yourself for several breaths: "I deserve this time to unwind."

MODIFICATIONS

- Ensure you are comfortable in this series by experimenting with the thickness of the blanket folds for your head support in Thread the Needle and under your chest in Supported Backbend.

- In Supported Bridge, try different heights of the block or use a rolled blanket under the sacrum.

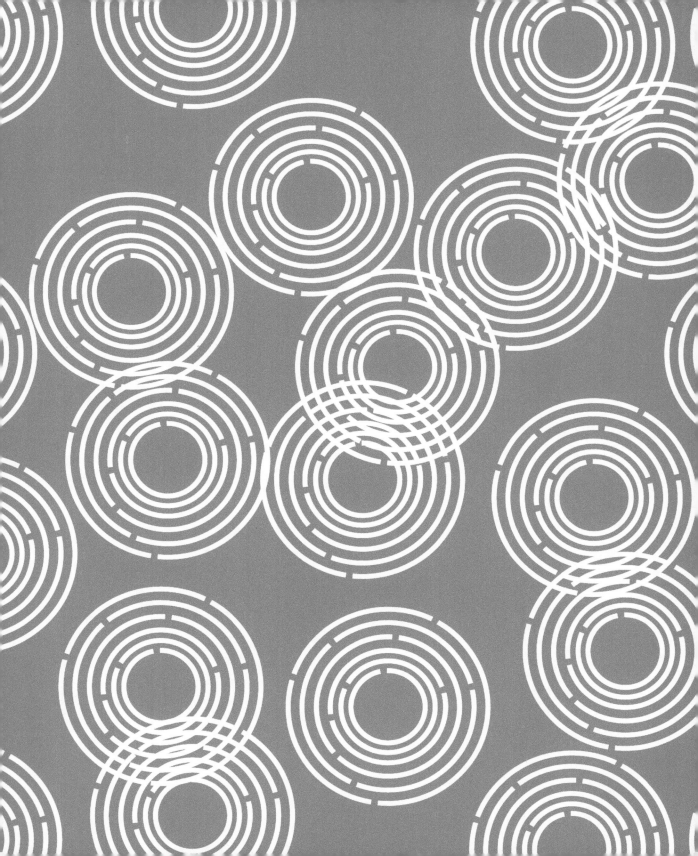

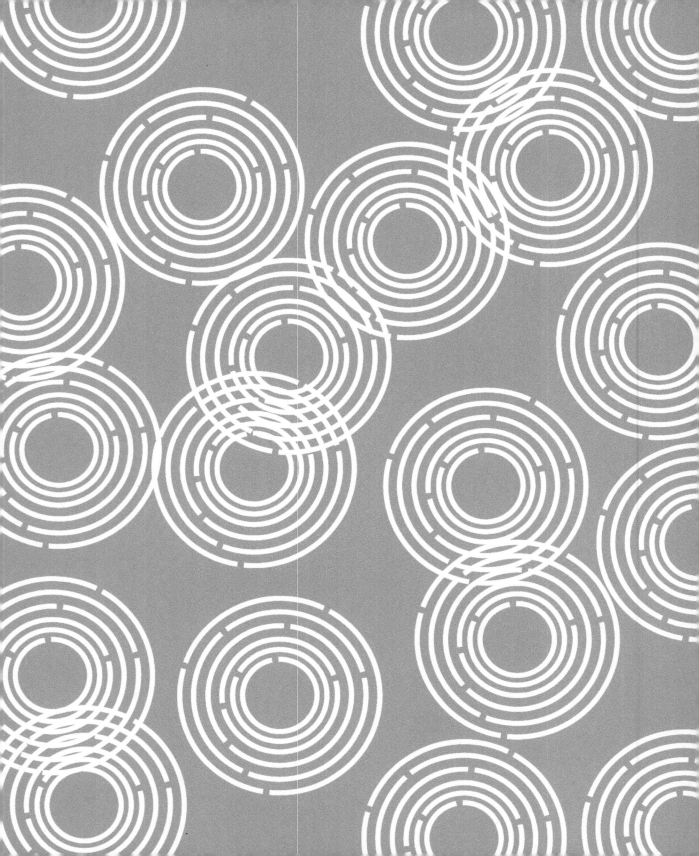

CHAPTER THREE

Lower-Body Poses and Sequences

The poses and sequences in this chapter address common issues and conditions of the lower body. Keep in mind that the yogic approach acknowledges the wholeness of our human system: mind, body, and breath. For example, as we move our legs through the Leg Stretch series (see page 143), our hips also receive healing motion and release. Further, although the target area in this chapter is the lower body, being mindful of our spinal alignment and postural awareness will help us breathe more fully. Breathing completely and with intention, and practicing the affirmations included with the sequences, will calm the mind, change our relationship to pain, and release stress in the lower body. The poses that target a variety of conditions. The stretching, restorative, and yin poses unwind the tension and guarding in our muscles that occur when we experience pain. Other poses build strength for recovery and prevention.

After the poses, there are five themed sequences. Each features three of the lower-body poses. Yoga emphasizes consistent practice, and just three poses can be the exact motivation to practice on a regular basis. You may decide to combine two sequences and practice six poses on some days, and on other days, you may find that one or two is all you need. Do what is best for you. And remember that consistency is key.

Hips, Glutes, and Pelvis

Bookmark this page! Each pose and sequence refers to different physical areas and muscle groups shown in this illustration.

iliopsoas (psoas major and iliascus) deep muscle stretching from the lumbar vertebrae across the pelvis to the lesser trochanter of the femur

piriformis deep rotator of the hip joint

ABDUCTORS outer hip muscles

tensor fasciae latae (TFL) and iliotibial tract (IT) muscle on the lateral hip and fascia on the lateral outside of the thigh. Runs across the knee joint and inserts on the outside of the shinbone (tibia), stabilizing the hips and knees. It also works with its associated muscles, the hip abductors and quadriceps, to extend, abduct, and laterally rotate the hip.

ADDUCTORS inner thigh and hip muscles

GLUTEALS muscles on the back of the hips— gluteus maximus (extends hip), gluteus medius and minimus (hip stabilizers, rotators, and abductors)

pelvic floor (supports pelvic floor organs, stabilizes connecting joints, aids in urinary, fecal, and sexual functions)

HAMSTRINGS (knee flexion and hip extension)

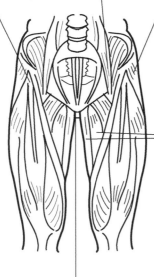
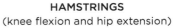

KNEES-TO-CHEST POSE

PHYSICAL AREAS TARGETED: erector spinae, quadratus lumborum (see page 69), hip flexors, gluteal group

BODY AND MIND AREAS RELIEVED: lower-back tightness and pain, hip tension, stress, sluggish digestion, shallow breathing

Knees-to-Chest Pose offers all levels of practitioners simple muscular tension relief, particularly in the lower back and hips. Your breath and movement are coordinated, and the respiratory diaphragm is safely stimulated to support your breathing capacity. You will experience how the movements in the pelvis affect your entire spine. The tactile feedback of the floor under your back and hips will remind you of the pelvic/spine movement relationship in other poses, such as Cat/Cow (see page 40) and seated Mountain Pose (see page 33).

COMMON CONDITIONS ADDRESSED

- Anxiety
- Breathing difficulty
- Digestive disorders
- Lower-back pain
- Overall tension and stress
- Sacroiliac joint pain

PROPS NEEDED: BLANKET (OPTIONAL), CHAIR (OPTIONAL)

Inhale.

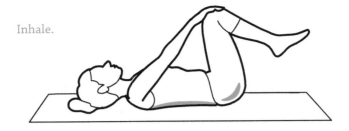

Exhale.

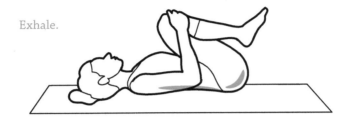

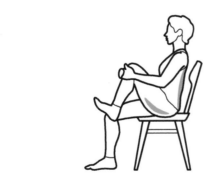

SEATED VARIATION: Keep the spine long and the jaw relaxed.

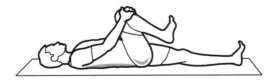

ONE-LEG VARIATION: Keep the lengthened heel pressing forward as you bring the opposite knee to the chest. Circle the bent knee leg in the hip joint if you wish.

1. Recline on your back with knees bent and feet on the floor, hip distance apart. If your chin is jutting toward the ceiling, place a blanket under the head and neck before proceeding.

2. Lift both feet off the floor. Place your right hand on your right knee and your left hand on your left knee.

3. On the inhale, draw your knees away from the chest, stacking them over the hip joints. Feel space at the lumbar spine without overarching your lower back. Your elbows will straighten.

4. On the exhale, bring your legs toward your chest and feel your lower back flatten to the floor. Let your elbows bend out.

5. Repeat 5 to 10 times at your own pace. Continue to synchronize your breathing, inhaling when your knees are over the hip joints, and exhaling when you hug your knees toward your chest.

6. To come out, release your feet to the floor and enjoy the effects of the pose.

TIPS

- Keep the jaw relaxed.

- Experiment by moving both knees in different directions (one clockwise and one counterclockwise) or imagining you are tracing the numbers of a clock on the ceiling with both knees moving in the same direction. Feel the massage of the lower back and hips.

MODIFICATIONS

- If you are unable to come to the floor, practice the chair modification. From seated Mountain Pose (see page 33), draw your knees toward your chest, one at a time, and keep the spine long. Maintain for 5 to 10 breaths.

- You can also try lying on your back and hugging one knee in at a time. The bottom leg can have a bent or straight knee.

RECLINED PIGEON

PHYSICAL AREAS TARGETED: piriformis and other deep rotators, quadratus lumborum (see page 69)

BODY AND MIND AREAS RELIEVED: tight hips, poor circulation, hip pain from pregnancy (see seated variation), stress, anxiety

Reclined Pigeon, sometimes known as Figure Four pose, is a versatile stretch of the lateral rotators of the hip. Tightness in the rotator (piriformis) can compress the sciatic nerve and cause hip and leg tingling or pain. Sitting too much, overdoing athletic endeavors, or hip pressure from pregnancy can cause hip discomfort or pain. There is a version of this pose for everyone, and yogis find universal relief in lengthening the muscles of the hips.

COMMON CONDITIONS ADDRESSED

- Hip stiffness from athletic endeavors
- Hip stiffness from sitting too much
- Piriformis syndrome
- Sciatic pain
- Shortened deep hip rotators

PROPS NEEDED: BLANKET (OPTIONAL), CHAIR (OPTIONAL)

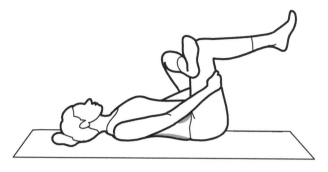

Maintain length in the spine and keep the top foot flexed.

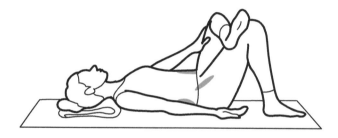

Gently press the top leg away to carefully deepen the stretch.

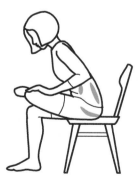

SEATED VARIATION: Keep the head in line with the rest of the spine and the bottom foot and leg stable in seated Mountain Pose.

1. Recline on your back with knees bent and feet on the floor, hip distance apart. If your chin is jutting toward the ceiling, place a blanket under the head and neck before proceeding.

2. Hug your right knee into your chest, then rotate that leg from the hip and place the right ankle above the left knee. Keep your right foot flexed, not pointed.

3. Throughout this pose, keep your sacrum on the floor to avoid rounding the back and to maintain the natural curve of the spine. Keep breathing gently as you experience a stretch and lengthening deep in the right hip.

4. Lift the left leg off the ground and carry the right leg with it. Thread your right hand into the window of space between the legs and hold the back of the left thigh with both hands. Alternatively, you can hold the shin of the left leg.

5. Continue to breathe, and experiment with gently pressing the bottom leg toward you and the top leg away from you while maintaining spinal length.

6. After 6 to 10 breaths, release both legs to the floor as one unit, then uncross the right ankle from the left leg.

7. Repeat this pose with the other side of your body.

TIPS

- If you are unable to lift the lower leg off the floor (step 4), you can still experience hip opening by keeping the bottom foot on the floor.

- Maintain relaxation in your jaw and face.

- After you stretch one side, observe how the hips feel different from each other before proceeding to the other side.

- Feel free to straighten the bottom leg toward the ceiling and add ankle circles.

MODIFICATION

Practice the seated version if lying on the floor isn't possible or if you are pregnant. In seated Mountain Pose (see page 33), sit toward the edge of your chair, draw the right knee to the chest with your hands, and rotate the right hip to place the right ankle above the left knee. Keep the left leg in seated Mountain Pose as you slowly hinge forward from the hip. Avoid jutting your chin out. Maintain the pose for several breaths as you hinge back up, take the right leg off the leg, and repeat on the other side.

CHAIR POSE

PHYSICAL AREAS TARGETED: quadriceps (see page 133), gluteal muscles, hip rotators and abductors, adductor group

BODY AND MIND AREAS RELIEVED: weak quadriceps, tight and weak gluteal muscles, tight and weak pelvic floor muscles, restricted breathing, decreased confidence

Chair Pose, also known as Powerful Pose, increases muscle and bone strength in your feet, ankles, calves, hips, lower back, and legs. In this pose, you're also activating your back and abdominal muscles. Chair Pose maintains your ability to move from a seated position to a standing one. This can be compromised if you are recovering from an illness, have sedentary habits, have experienced age-related muscle loss, are carrying additional weight, or are pregnant. Chair Pose cultivates mental fortitude for improved self-confidence, focus, willpower, and calm as you challenge yourself physically.

COMMON CONDITIONS ADDRESSED

- General lower body and back weakness from a sedentary lifestyle
- Imbalanced inner and outer leg muscles
- Lower-back pain
- Pelvic floor muscle imbalances
- Sacroiliac joint pain
- Shallow breathing

PROPS NEEDED: BLOCK OR BALL (OPTIONAL)

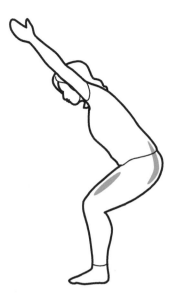

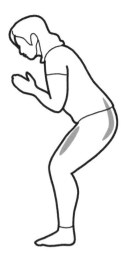

Knees are stacked over the ankles, not
past the toes, the spine is long, the
pelvis is neutral, and the tops of the
hips are in line with the bottom ribs.

You can choose to place your hands
together at the heart.

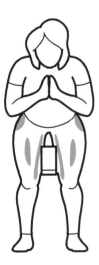

Place a block between your legs to remind you to
engage the adductors (inner thigh muscles).

1. From Mountain Pose (see page 33), inhale, bend your knees, and lower your hips behind your body as though you are about to sit in a chair.

2. Check your knees to make sure they aren't moving past your toes.

3. Track the knees physically and energetically toward the middle toes of the feet. Think "knees over ankles."

4. Press slightly more weight into your heels to engage your back-of-the-body muscles. Feel the gluteal muscles elongate. You will also engage your quadriceps (thigh muscles).

5. Engage the core muscles of the low belly, preventing the pelvis from rotating forward too much.

6. Breathe with the full 360-degree breath (see page 13) for 5 to 10 breaths. Stay calm yet focused and determined.

7. On an exhale, press into the heels and engage the lower body. Feel the pelvic floor lift in and up on the exhale.

TIPS

- Imagine your bottom ribs are aligned with the top of your pelvis. Feel your core engage.

- Maintain a neutral lumbar spine. Avoid overarching or rounding the back or tilting the pelvis too far forward or backward.

- You can place a block or a ball between the inner thighs as a tactile reminder to engage the adductor muscles of the upper legs.

- To improve strength, experiment with counting breaths, increasing your time in the pose with every other practice. For example, start with 3 breaths and work up to 5 breaths.

MODIFICATIONS

- Experiment with upper-body arm positions. Options can include Cactus Arms (see page 56), prayer position, or arms next to the ears.

- If you have tender knees or a knee injury, modify with the High Chair version of the pose, pictured. For the High Chair Pose, lower your hips only slightly as though sitting on a high stool, and bend your knees minimally, just until you feel your thighs engage.

TREE POSE

PHYSICAL AREAS TARGETED: gluteus medius, tensor fasciae latae, hip flexors, quadriceps, adductor group, iliopsoas

BODY AND MIND AREAS RELIEVED: tight hips, weak gluteal muscles, weak leg muscles, unsteady balance, osteoporosis, decreased confidence, weak ankles

Tree Pose is a well-known, one-leg balance pose. There are several variations, so you can do this posture regardless of your experience or physical abilities. Tree Pose increases lower-body strength, confidence, postural awareness, hip and ankle flexibility, and balance. This pose also cultivates the capacity to breathe and concentrate, illustrating how mindful presence can support physical balance. Practicing Tree Pose creates a standing meditative focus and dials down stress.

COMMON CONDITIONS ADDRESSED

- Hip tightness
- Lower-body weakness
- Osteoporosis
- Poor concentration
- Sciatica
- Unsteady balance

PROPS NEEDED: WALL OR CHAIR (OPTIONAL)

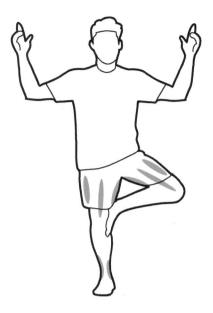

CACTUS ARMS VARIATION:
Keep the gaze steady and the energy
at the midline of the body.

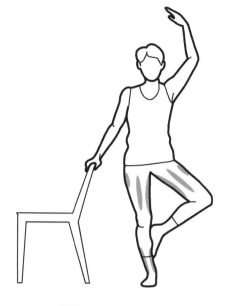

CHAIR VARIATION:
Practice next to a support for confidence and safety.

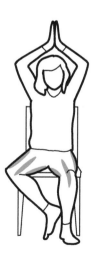

SEATED VARIATION:
Practice the pose seated if standing
balance is unavailable to you.

1. Stand steadily in Mountain Pose (see page 33) before shifting your weight to your right foot. You can begin the pose with your hands on your hips.

2. Rotate your left hip externally so the knee points more to your left. Place your left heel on the inner lower leg, keeping your left toes on the ground and the right foot mindfully connected to the earth. Keep your hips stable and as even as possible. Magnetize the left and right side of the body to the midline so you feel strong, like the core of a tree trunk.

3. Depending on the flexibility of your left hip and your current balance ability, you can raise the heel of the left foot manually and place it below or above the right knee joint. Do not rest the heel against the knee joint.

4. You can place your arms in various positions. Options include your hands at your hips, your hands in prayer position in front of your heart, your arms stretched out to the sides, Cactus Arms, or your arms raised up to the sky with hands apart or palms joined.

5. After several breaths, slowly come out of the pose and pause in Mountain Pose before practicing on the other side.

TIPS

- Any version of Downward-Facing Dog (see page 70) is a good symmetrical follow-up pose.

- Lengthen the top of the head toward the sky for postural stability awareness.

- You are balancing in this pose, so don't worry if your body isn't static. The ankle might be moving slightly, you might sway, and you might find it's easier to balance on one leg than the other. All of this is normal.

- Experiment with breath counting to see if you can increase your time in the pose with regular practice.

MODIFICATIONS

- Practice with your fingers near or on a support, such as a wall or chair, to build confidence or if you are pregnant.

- If you are unable to stand, practice seated Tree Pose while still cultivating focus and upper-body strength.

VICTORY/GODDESS SQUAT

PHYSICAL AREAS TARGETED: quadriceps (see page 133), pelvic floor, adductor group gastrocnemius (see page 154)

BODY AND MIND AREAS RELIEVED: weak quadriceps, tight or weak adductors, shallow breath, pelvic floor tightness, anxiety, fear

Victory/Goddess Squat is an empowering lower-body strengthening pose. Whether you practice it statically or dynamically, it enhances inner fortitude, physical strength, and flexibility. Variations are available for every point of your healing journey. You can coordinate pelvic and respiratory diaphragmatic breathing as you move in and out of this symmetrical pose. If you are in the latter weeks of pregnancy, do not squat deeply. Consult with your medical provider if you recently had knee or hip surgery.

COMMON CONDITIONS ADDRESSED

- Gluteal muscle and sacroiliac joint imbalances
- Lack of leg strength
- Pelvic floor muscle imbalances
- Stiff or tight hips

- Weak muscles around the knees

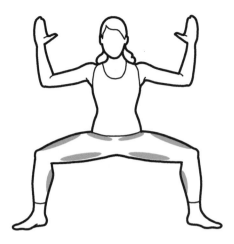

Align the knees over the ankles toward the smaller toes of the feet.
Keep the core strong. This pose is shown with Cactus Arms.

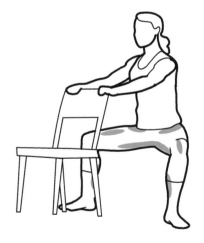

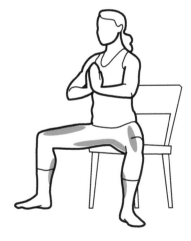

CHAIR VARIATION:
Be sure the chair is stable, and squat
comfortably, practicing safe knee
alignment.

SEATED VARIATION:
Sit toward the edge of the chair.
Take any comfortable arm position.

1. Facing the long side of your mat, step your feet as wide as you comfortably can.

2. Rotate your toes toward the front corners of the mat and feel your hips rotating out in coordination.

3. Bend your knees and take one small test squat. Check that your knees are energizing toward the middle toes of the feet and not buckling in toward the midline of your body. Adjust your stance as needed. Feel your hips move straight down to the floor and keep your spine and core muscles strong.

4. You can place your arms and hands in various positions: prayer position, Cactus Arms (see page 56), Eagle Arms (see page 59), or on your thighs to feel the work in the quadriceps.

5. Static version: Squat more deeply in the pose and hold for 3 or more breaths. Work up to 10 breaths over time.

6. Dynamic version: Inhale into the pelvic floor and respiratory diaphragm as you squat, and on your exhale, straighten the knees and feel the pelvic floor contract in and up as the abdominals contract. Repeat 4 to 6 times.

7. To come out of the pose, walk your feet back to Mountain Pose (see page 33). If you'd like, follow up with Dancer Pose (see page 134) for a nice stretch of your quadriceps.

TIPS

- Keep your knees over your ankles; do not let them move past your toes.

- Mentally affirm "I am becoming stronger" and "I am capable."

MODIFICATIONS

- Chair variation: Use a chair for balance and stability. Making sure the chair is stable on the floor or mat, lightly hold on to the chair in front of you instead of taking the arm position variations.

- Seated variation: Sit on the edge of a chair while maintaining lower-body knee alignment. You can benefit from the pose even if it is currently challenging to balance or to bear too much weight in the lower body.

WARRIOR I

PHYSICAL AREAS TARGETED: quadriceps and hamstrings (see page 133), gluteus maximus (hip extensor), gluteus medius and gluteus minimus (hip rotators and stabilizers), abductors, psoas, adductor group, tensor fasciae latae, hip flexors, erector spinae (see page 69), gastrocnemius (see page 154)

BODY AND MIND AREAS RELIEVED: tight hip flexors, weak quadriceps, tight gluteal muscles, unsteady balance, restricted breathing, low energy

Warrior I is an essential standing yoga pose. A variation of lunging, it creates opening in the hip joint tissues of the back leg. Simultaneously, the front leg is engaged, which strengthens the quadriceps muscles and protects the knee joint. Safely challenging the legs and hips in a wider stance helps prepare you for walking and stair climbing and prevents you from shuffling. This pose strengthens the mind and body.

COMMON CONDITIONS ADDRESSED

- Hip tightness
- Lower-body weakness
- Osteoporosis
- Unsteady balance
- Walking stride issues

PROPS NEEDED: TABLE OR CHAIR (OPTIONAL), BLANKET (OPTIONAL)

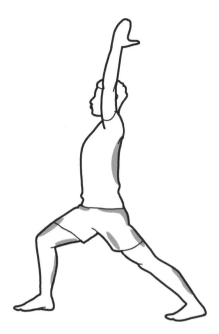

Make sure your front knee is stacked over your ankle. Keep your gaze and breathing steady and feel the inner lift of the spine.

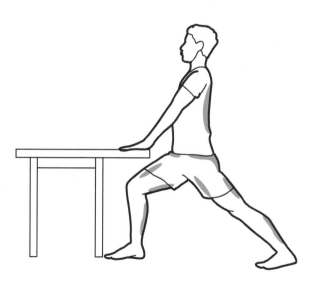

TABLE VARIATION: Practice with your hands on a table, countertop, or chair if balance is a challenge.

1. Facing the short end of the mat, step your left foot as far back to the rear of the mat as you comfortably can, keeping your heels hip distance apart. Make sure both feet are on the mat.

2. Point the left toes toward the left side of the mat, keeping the heel on the mat.

3. Bend the right knee, keeping it aligned over your right ankle, and point the knee energetically toward the middle toes of the right foot.

4. Move your spine in, forward, and up. The ribs can move slightly in front of the pelvis to lift out of the lumbar spine and avoid a compressed feeling.

5. You can take several different arm positions, including raising your arms alongside your ears with the palms facing the midline of the body, Cactus Arms (see page 56), or hands on hips.

6. To practice the pose dynamically, bend and straighten the front knee 2 or 3 times while breathing, and then stay for 3 to 5 breaths to build strength.

7. To release the pose, relax the arms and step the left foot forward to the right foot. Pause in Mountain Pose and notice the difference between your two sides.

8. Repeat on the other side.

TIPS

- Place your hands on your pelvis and adjust the back pelvis slightly forward and the front pelvis slightly back so you have a sense of squaring. Note that the pelvis will not be perfectly squared forward.

- Keep your stance as wide as your hips to feel a sense of stability.

- If your back heel doesn't go to the floor, support it with a rolled-up blanket, keep it slightly off the floor, or take a slightly wider stance.

MODIFICATION

Practice with your hands on a table or chair if balance is a challenge.

LEGS-UP-THE-WALL POSE

PHYSICAL AREAS TARGETED: hamstrings (see page 133), pelvic floor (see page 133), psoas

BODY AND MIND AREAS RELIEVED: swollen feet, cramping, poor circulation, jaw clenching, back pain, tight chest, anxiety

Legs-Up-the-Wall Pose is a gentle, accessible restorative inversion that facilitates the relaxation response and counteracts the effects of stress on the body, mind, and spirit. You will redistribute body fluids and relieve pressure on the legs. There is also support for the torso, head, and arms, so you don't need to engage muscle tone to practice this shape. You can relax even more by placing an eye bag or a cloth over your eyes. If you have glaucoma or uncontrolled high blood pressure, check with your physician before engaging in this pose; it may be contraindicated because the blood pressure temporarily rises as you go into the pose, before downregulating.

COMMON CONDITIONS ADDRESSED

- Anxiety
- General fatigue
- Insomnia
- Jet lag
- Menstrual cramps, perimeno-pause, and menopause
- Pelvic floor tightness
- Stress
- Varicose veins

PROPS NEEDED: BLANKET(S) (OPTIONAL), CLOTH OR EYE BAG (OPTIONAL), CHAIR (OPTIONAL)

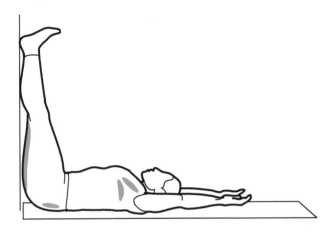

Hips flat on the ground or on a blanket, forehead and chin level
with the ceiling (chin not jutting out).

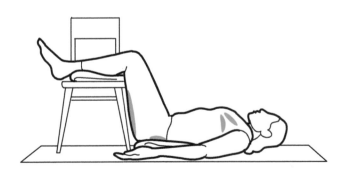

CHAIR VARIATION: Optional blankets under hips and
calves. Pelvis is level. Adjust the chair so your knees are at
a right angle.

1. Sit with your right or left hip next to the wall. You can bring the short end of your mat to the wall if you want to be on the mat.

2. With your hands braced on the floor behind you, lean your torso back slightly and swing your legs up the wall. Your distance from the wall will depend partly on your current hamstring flexibility, so take time to adjust your hips so they are as close to the wall as possible.

3. Make sure the sacrum is flat on the floor or supported by a blanket.

4. Before relaxing into the pose, raise your head and make sure your body looks symmetrical. Adjust accordingly.

5. Your arms can be by your sides, palms up, or in Cactus Arms (see page 56).

6. Relax and breathe in the pose. Hold for 5 to 20 minutes.

7. To come out of the pose, slide your heels, one at a time, down the wall. With your knees bent, roll over to either side and rest for several breaths.

8. Use your arm strength to press up slowly back to seated.

9. Enjoy the sense of renewal and calm. Spend a few moments in your choice of meditation.

TIPS

- If you would like your hips on a blanket, set the blanket about 8 inches from the wall, across the mat, before swinging your legs up the wall.

- If your hamstrings are tight, it's fine if the backs of the legs aren't completely touching the wall. You can even bend the knees slightly.

- Slide the heels down and up the wall one at a time if your feet begin to tingle, then resume the pose.

- Place a blanket under the head and neck if your chin is jutting up toward the ceiling.

MODIFICATION

Practice the legs-on-a-chair variation if you are still working on flexibility or if Legs-Up-the-Wall is impractical or uncomfortable. Gather your blanket and eye cover if you would like. Sit on the floor or blanket with your right or left hip in front of a chair with the seat facing you. Bracing your arms behind you, turn your hips and place your calves on the chair. Take time to adjust and ensure that your pelvis is flat on the floor or on the blanket. Adjust the chair so your knees are bent at a right angle. Relax in the pose for 5 to 20 minutes. When it's time to come out of the pose, bend your knees, roll onto your side, and rest for a few breaths before sitting up.

Thighs and Knees

Bookmark this page! Each pose and sequence refers to different physical areas and muscle groups shown in this illustration.

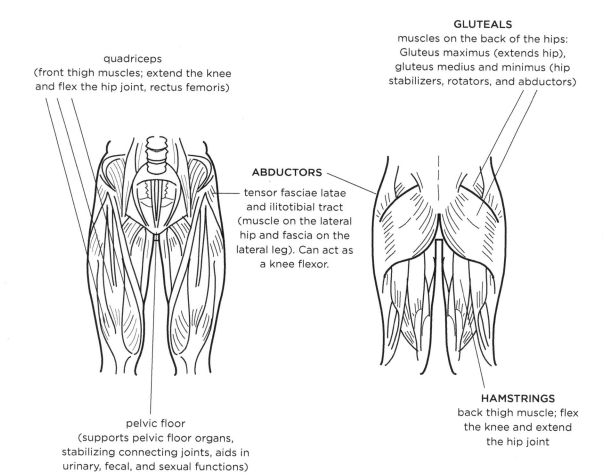

GLUTEALS
muscles on the back of the hips:
Gluteus maximus (extends hip),
gluteus medius and minimus (hip
stabilizers, rotators, and abductors)

quadriceps
(front thigh muscles; extend the knee
and flex the hip joint, rectus femoris)

ABDUCTORS

tensor fasciae latae
and ilitotibial tract
(muscle on the lateral
hip and fascia on the
lateral leg). Can act as
a knee flexor.

HAMSTRINGS
back thigh muscle; flex
the knee and extend
the hip joint

pelvic floor
(supports pelvic floor organs,
stabilizing connecting joints, aids in
urinary, fecal, and sexual functions)

DANCER POSE

PHYSICAL AREAS TARGETED: quadriceps, hip flexors, erector spinae (see page 69)

BODY AND MIND AREAS RELIEVED: tight hip flexors, stiff thighs, weak or overly tight core muscles, stiff knees, tight chest and shoulders

Although it is crucial to maintain and increase strength in the quadriceps (thighs), you can become tight and contracted from overworking this muscle group. One of the main jobs of the quadriceps is to extend the knee joint. Restricted range of motion in the quadriceps can cause discomfort when bending and flexing the knee joint. This pose can also address tight hip flexors, a common result of inactivity, as well as quadriceps flexibility. Check with your health care provider before engaging in Dancer Pose if you recently had knee surgery.

COMMON CONDITIONS ADDRESSED

- Ill effects of too much sitting
- Lack of focus and concentration
- Muscle imbalances between the thighs and hamstrings
- Overuse injuries from athletic endeavors
- Unsteady balance
- Weak muscles and bones in the legs

PROPS NEEDED: WALL, CHAIR, OR TABLE; STRAP (OPTIONAL)

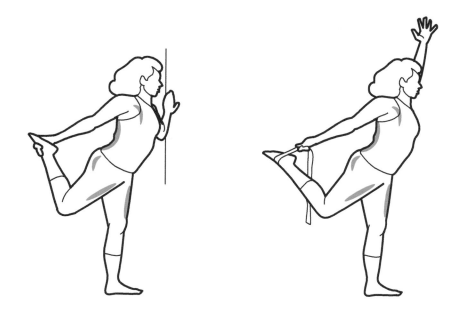

Keep the spine moving in and up and avoid letting the knee splay out.

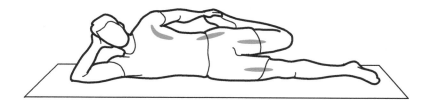

FLOOR VARIATION: Rest your head on your hand
or upper arm. Keep your hips and knees parallel.

1. Stand in Mountain Pose (see page 33) near a wall, chair, or table for safety and balance.

2. Bend your left knee and bring your heel toward your left gluteal muscle. Grab your left foot or ankle with your left hand. Lightly hold the support with your right hand, or place the hand on your hip. Maintain steady breath and keep the shoulders relaxed away from your ears.

3. Keep your knees and thighs as close together as your body will allow, preventing the left knee from angling out to the side.

4. Gently press the hips slightly forward as the bent knee moves slightly backward and feel the thigh stretch extending into the hip flexors.

5. If you would like to expand the pose, begin to draw the heel away from the left buttock, lengthening the spine in and up for a gentle backbend. Practice this version near a wall for safety and confidence.

6. After 5 or more breaths, slowly release the foot and stand in Mountain Pose. Note the difference between the two sides of the body.

7. Repeat on the other side.

TIPS

- Continue to engage your core muscles throughout the pose while lengthening the spine.

- Move slowly and gently if you have knee arthritis or any other knee issues.

- If you are not able to grab your ankle, clasp your pant leg or loop a strap around your foot.

- Dancer Pose is a wonderful counterpose to Chair Pose (see page 117) or Warrior II (see page 137).

MODIFICATION

If standing is a challenge, modify this pose by lying on your side on the floor. Practice steps 2 through 4, making sure to stretch both legs. You can rest your head on your hand with your elbow bent or on your forearm with a straight elbow.

WARRIOR II

PHYSICAL AREAS TARGETED: quadriceps, hamstrings, tensor fasciae latae, hip flexors and abductors (see page 110), iliotibial tract, gluteus medius (see page 110)

BODY AND MIND AREAS RELIEVED: weak legs, impaired breathing, weak core, tight inner thighs, pregnancy discomforts, lack of mental empowerment

Warrior II is a well-known, physically and mentally empowering pose. In a wider-than-normal stance, the leg muscles engage for strength and balance. The hips receive a nice opening. Various upper-body arm positions are available to enhance your strength and open your chest for optimal breathing. You can practice this pose statically or dynamically. Steady determination and ease are cultivated.

COMMON CONDITIONS ADDRESSED

- Back pain
- Decreased mental and physical fortitude
- Lower-body muscle tightness
- Lower-body muscle weakness
- Osteoporosis
- Restricted breathing
- Tight hips
- Tight inner thighs

PROPS NEEDED: CHAIR (OPTIONAL)

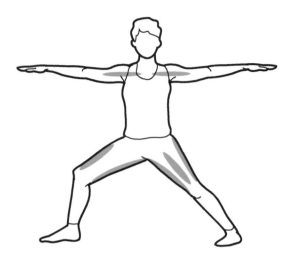

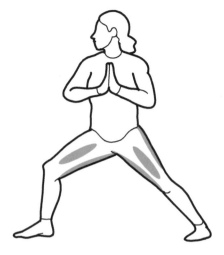

Knee joint does not move past
toes. Back heel and toes are turned
slightly in.

Practice with prayer hands if you are
experiencing any shoulder restrictions.

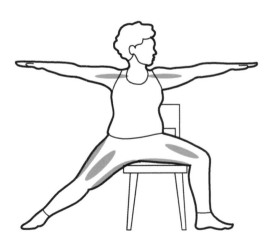

SEATED VARIATION: Sit toward the edge of the chair with pelvis
supported. Use the same leg alignment as the standing version.

1. Facing the long side of the mat, step your feet as wide as you comfortably can.

2. Turn your right leg to the right so the toes of the right foot are parallel with the long edge of the mat. Turn your left toes slightly toward the midline of the body. Feel the rotation of the foot originating from the left hip.

3. Look at your feet and align the front heel with the back heel. Your legs and feet are the foundation of this pose.

4. Inhale and extend your arms out alongside your body, raising them to shoulder height, palms facing down. Softly gaze over the middle finger of your right hand and relax your shoulders away from your ears.

5. As your right knee bends, feel your hips lower straight down. Keep your core muscles engaged, your jaw soft, and your breath steady. Remain in the pose for 5 to 10 breaths.

6. To come out of the pose, relax the arms and straighten the front knee. Pause for a few breaths before repeating the pose on the left side of the body.

TIPS

- Energize your bent knee toward the smaller toes of the feet and stack the knee over the ankle. Feel your ribs stacking over the top of the pelvis so you don't lean too far forward or backward.

- Keep pressing the heel of the straight leg into the floor.

- The bent knee does not have to bend completely.

- Do not overly widen the legs if you start to feel imbalanced.

MODIFICATIONS

- If you have any neck issues, look forward instead of sideways over your hand.

- If you have any shoulder issues, practice with your hands in prayer position or at your hip.

- If standing is difficult or if you are in the last few weeks of pregnancy, practice the seated variation. To practice with a chair, sit toward the edge of the chair and adjust to align the back and front heels with each other. Modify the position of your hips so you can feel support under the thigh of the bent knee. Practice steps 4 through 6. Come out of the pose and pause in seated Mountain Pose (see page 33) before taking the second side.

SIDE-ANGLE POSE

PHYSICAL AREAS TARGETED: quadriceps, hamstrings, gluteal muscles (see page 110), tensor fasciae latae, hip flexors (see page 110), serratus anterior (see page 68), obliques (see page 69)

BODY AND MIND AREAS RELIEVED: digestive disorders, low back pain, osteoporosis, sciatica, overall mental and physical weakness, menstrual discomfort

Side-Angle Pose strengthens and increases flexibility in your legs. You will experience increased hip mobility and improved balance even though both feet are on the ground. Additionally, the upper body lengthens, which creates more room for your entire breath. Side-Angle Pose is another versatile essential standing pose that improves inner and outer feelings of empowerment as your strength increases.

COMMON CONDITIONS ADDRESSED

- Balancing issues
- Breathing restrictions
- Fatigue
- Inflexibility
- Osteoporosis
- Weak knees

PROPS NEEDED: CHAIR (OPTIONAL), WALL (OPTIONAL)

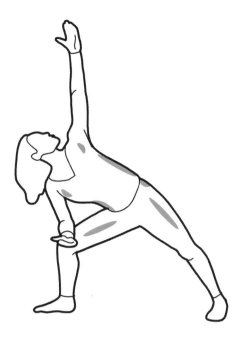

Keep the spine and both sides of the torso long. Stack the upper wrist over the shoulder and look up only if it feels comfortable to you.

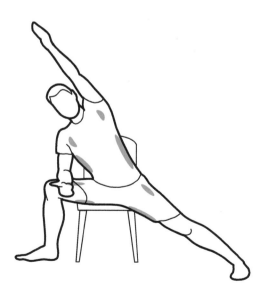

SEATED VARIATION: Modify the upper arm position if lengthening alongside the ear is restrictive for the shoulder.

1. Facing the long side of the mat, step your feet as wide as you comfortably can.

2. Turn your right leg to the right so the toes of the right foot are parallel with the long edge of the mat. Turn your left toes slightly toward the midline of the body. Feel the rotation of the toes from the left hip.

3. Look at your feet and align the front heel with the back heel. Your legs and feet are the foundation of this pose.

4. Bend your right knee so it is directly over your ankle.

5. Place your right forearm on your right thigh. Avoid sinking into the forearm and shoulder by engaging your core and lengthening the spine and both sides of the torso.

6. Lengthen your left arm up to the sky so the left wrist aligns over the left shoulder.

7. Look up toward the left thumb as you feel the left side of the chest and the tissues around the lungs start to open.

8. After 3 to 6 breaths, press strongly into the feet and engage the back body to come out of the pose.

9. Repeat on the left side.

10. Pause in Mountain Pose (see page 33) or practice Downward-Facing Dog (see page 70).

TIPS

- Anchor the back heel to a wall to enhance strength and balance.

- If you have neck restrictions, avoid looking up.

- Side-Angle Pose is a natural follow-up pose to Warrior II (see page 137).

MODIFICATIONS

- Practice the seated version if standing is difficult or if you are in the last few weeks of pregnancy. To practice with a chair, sit toward the edge of the chair and adjust to align your back and front heels with each other. Modify the position of your hips so you can feel support under the thigh of the bent knee. Practice steps 5 through 9.

- Various positions are available for your upper arm, depending on your shoulder flexibility. If you have shoulder restrictions, keep the back hand on your hip or waist.

LEG STRETCH #2 AND LEG STRETCH #3

PHYSICAL AREAS TARGETED: hamstrings, adductor group, tensor fasciae latae, iliotibial tract, pelvic floor (see page 110)

BODY AND MIND AREAS RELIEVED: tight hamstrings, tight hips, tight/weak pelvic floor, adductor and abductor tightness, back pain

Leg-stretch variations are a highly accessible yoga series for both beginners and seasoned practitioners. Over- or underuse of the leg and hip muscles can restrict movement, and these poses gently guide you through various positions to restore mobility. You can practice the series reclined or seated, and it is frequently used for overall strengthening and recovery after a long period of immobility. Your back is supported on the floor, so you won't feel the usual gravitational challenges when practicing an advanced standing variation. These two postures are the natural follow-ups to Leg Stretch #1 (see page 158).

COMMON CONDITIONS ADDRESSED

- Imbalanced walking or running gait
- Low confidence for standing poses
- Lower-body restrictions from sitting too much
- Tightness in iliotibial band from overuse
- Weak core muscles

PROPS NEEDED: YOGA STRAP, BLANKET (OPTIONAL), CHAIR (OPTIONAL)

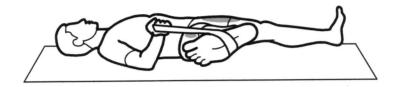

RECLINED LEG STRETCH #2 VARIATION: Keep the leg and hip of the nonstrapped leg stable by not letting it pop up. Align the ankle, knee, and hip joint as if you were standing upright.

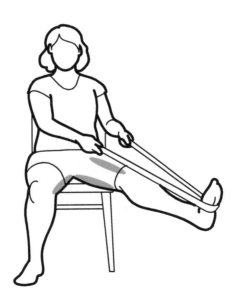

SEATED LEG STRETCH #2 VARIATION: Maintain relaxed shoulders and core strength as you guide the strapped leg open to your end range.

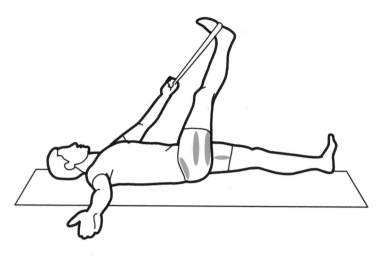

RECLINED LEG STRETCH #3 VARIATION: Cross the strapped leg over the midline of the body just enough to feel lengthening along the outer hip and leg line.

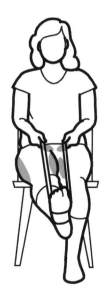

SEATED LEG STRETCH #3 VARIATION: Cross the leg over the midline of the body just enough to feel lengthening along the outer hip and thigh.

1. Recline on your back with both knees bent and heels hip distance apart.

2. Holding the strap with both hands, bring the right knee toward the chest and place the strap on the arch of the right foot.

3. Slowly straighten the right knee. Slide the left heel on the floor until the left leg is straight, toes facing the sky. Make sure the left hip, knee, and ankle are in alignment, as though you were standing on the floor.

4. Begin with Leg Stretch #1 (see page 158): Move the strapped right foot into any position that keeps the right knee straight without strain. If you are less flexible, the leg will move away from your upper body; if you are more flexible, the leg will move closer to the upper body.

5. Leg Stretch #2: With the strap in your right hand, rotate the right knee and hip away from the midline of the body and guide the right leg to the right side until you reach your end range. After 4 to 8 breaths, guide your leg back to #1, bend your knee, and release the strap from the foot. Pause, then repeat Leg Stretch #2 with the strap on the left leg.

6. Leg Stretch #3: From Leg Stretch #1 with the strap on the arch of the foot, hold the strap in your left hand and cross the right leg over the left side of the body until you feel lengthening along the outer line of the right hip and leg. Keep the right side of the pelvis stable; do not bring it along with the leg.

7. If you wish, stretch your right arm to the side and gaze to the ceiling or the right. After 4 to 8 breaths, guide your leg back to Leg Stretch #1, pause, and repeat Leg Stretch #3 with the strap on the arch of the left foot.

8. Bend your knee and release the strap. Pause or take Knees-to-Chest Pose (see page 111).

TIPS

- Place your hand on the hip of the nonstrapped leg to keep it stable in Leg Stretch #2.

- The strapped leg may shake a bit as you begin to gain flexibility. Over time, the shaking will subside. Back out of the stretch a bit as needed.

- Place a blanket under the head and neck if your chin is jutting too much toward the ceiling. Keep the upper back and shoulder blades connected to the floor as the chest remains open for your breath.

Practice the seated variation if reclining on the floor is currently difficult or you are more than three months pregnant. Sit toward the edge of the chair in seated Mountain Pose (see page 33). Perform the Leg Stretch series while maintaining joint alignment of the hip, knee, and ankle of the strapped leg.

RECLINED BOUND ANGLE

PHYSICAL AREAS TARGETED: adductor group, pelvic floor (see page 110), pectoralis muscles (see page 68)

BODY AND MIND AREAS RELIEVED: tight adductors, tight pectoralis muscles, restrictions or tightness in pelvic floor muscles, menstrual cramps, menopausal symptoms, mental and physical stress, anxiety

Reclined Bound Angle is a quintessential restorative pose. Gravity assists in unraveling tension in the inner thighs and pelvis. The pectoralis muscles in the chest can open to assist in the breathing for relaxation. You can get the benefits of this pose with minimal props, as shown in the illustrations. Even for those who are bedridden, bringing the soles of the feet together while reclined often releases overall stress and relaxes joint tension in the hips and inner thighs.

COMMON CONDITIONS ADDRESSED

- Difficulty breathing
- Lower-body circulatory restrictions
- Mental anxiety and stress
- Overall muscle tension
- Pelvic pain
- Pregnancy discomfort
- Sacroiliac joint imbalances
- Tight inner thigh muscles

PROPS NEEDED: BLANKET(S), BOLSTER AND BLOCK (OPTIONAL)

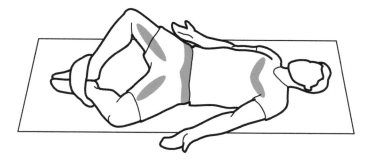

Heels are evenly aligned. In this "diamond" version, used if the hamstrings are less flexible, the heels are farther away from the hips.

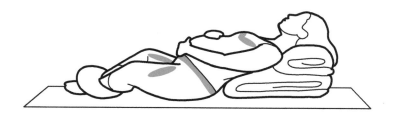

BOLSTER VARIATION: Modification for pregnancy or increased chest opening: The head and neck are supported, chin relaxed, chest open.

1. Roll a blanket into a tube and arrange it into a horseshoe shape.

2. With the horseshoe-shaped blanket and an optional folded blanket nearby, sit on your mat.

3. Bring the soles of the feet together evenly and rotate the hips and knees away from your body's midline.

4. Firmly place the horseshoe blanket around the tops of both ankles and tuck the ends of the blanket under your shins. Lie down on your mat.

5. Place the second blanket under the head and neck if your chin is jutting up toward the ceiling.

6. Breathe softly, relaxing the skin of your face, jaw, and forehead.

7. Allow gravity and time (a minimum of 5 minutes, maximum of 25 minutes) to release tension and stress.

8. To come out of the pose, place your hands on your outer thighs to help move your legs together. Roll to one side, pausing and breathing, and enjoy the effects of the practice.

TIPS

- If your knees are jutting up above your hips, slide your heels away from your hips to create the diamond-shaped version of the pose.

- Experiment with how close you can get your heels to your pelvis.

- Ensure that your heels are touching evenly. This will help align the hip and sacroiliac joints.

MODIFICATION

For pregnant women or for greater chest opening, take a bolster (or create one by rolling two yoga blankets together lengthwise) and place a block under it to create a ramp-like angle. Bring your hips to the edge of the bolster, and lie back with the support of your arms on either side. You can place your hands on your belly, your thighs, or the floor, palms up. This variation adds a greater chest opening.

BANANA POSE

PHYSICAL AREAS TARGETED: iliotibial tract, quadriceps, gluteus maximus (see page 110), intercostals, obliques (see page 69)

BODY AND MIND AREAS RELIEVED: tight hips, imbalanced quadriceps, knee pain, tight oblique muscles, spinal imbalances, imbalances on the lateral fascial lines of the body, digestion difficulties

Banana is a unique reclined yin pose that creates space in the often-neglected lateral lines of the body. The beauty of this shape is that you can practice it on the floor or even in bed. Repetitive overuse, a sedentary lifestyle, or moving your legs in only one direction (biking, walking, running) can cause imbalances in the hips and pelvic floor. This side stretch also opens the muscles and tissues between the ribs (intercostals), which support your 360-degree breath.

COMMON CONDITIONS ADDRESSED

- Breathing restrictions
- Foot misalignment
- Iliotibial band syndrome
- Knee misalignment
- Menstrual cramps

- Overuse of lower-body muscles in one direction
- Stiff lower body from a sedentary lifestyle
- Stress

PROPS NEEDED: NONE

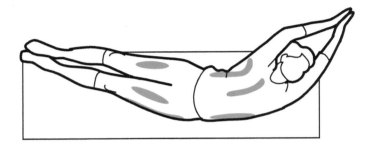

Keep your hips stationary as the upper and lower
body move to one side. Modify the arms overhead as
described in step 2.

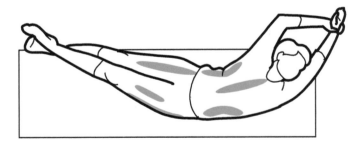

Cross the outer ankle over the inner ankle to intensify the stretch.

1. Rest on your back with your legs together.

2. Bring your arms overhead, clasping your hands, wrists, or elbows. If you don't have enough shoulder flexibility, keep your arms parallel.

3. Without moving your hips, move your feet and then your upper body to the right. Pause when you begin to feel sensation on the left side of the body. After several breaths, you may be able to move the upper and lower body to the right even more.

4. After 2 to 4 minutes, slowly bring your upper and lower body to the center. Lie still or take Knees-to-Chest Pose (see page 111).

5. Repeat, moving your upper and lower body to the left.

TIPS

- Observe and honor the differences between the two sides of the body.

- Be sure to keep your hips still when you move your upper and lower body to the same side. Moving your hips compromises the opening on the other side of the body.

MODIFICATION

For the most intense lateral stretch, cross the outer ankle over the inner ankle.

Calves, Ankles, and Feet

Bookmark this page! Each pose and sequence refers to different physical areas and muscle groups shown in this illustration.

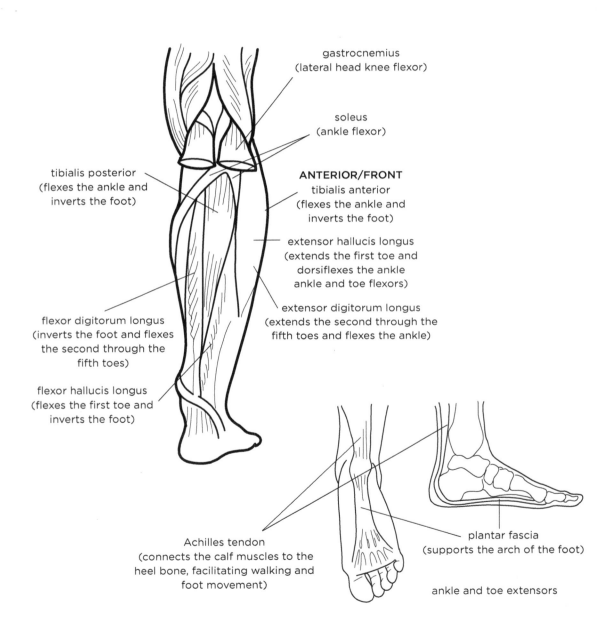

gastrocnemius
(lateral head knee flexor)

soleus
(ankle flexor)

ANTERIOR/FRONT
tibialis anterior
(flexes the ankle and
inverts the foot)

extensor hallucis longus
(extends the first toe and
dorsiflexes the ankle
ankle and toe flexors)

extensor digitorum longus
(extends the second through the
fifth toes and flexes the ankle)

tibialis posterior
(flexes the ankle and
inverts the foot)

flexor digitorum longus
(inverts the foot and flexes
the second through the
fifth toes)

flexor hallucis longus
(flexes the first toe and
inverts the foot)

Achilles tendon
(connects the calf muscles to the
heel bone, facilitating walking and
foot movement)

plantar fascia
(supports the arch of the foot)

ankle and toe extensors

HEEL LIFTS WITH ARM WAVES

PHYSICAL AREAS TARGETED: plantar fascia, Achilles tendon, soleus, gastrocnemius

BODY AND MIND AREAS RELIEVED: sore feet, tight ankles, stiff Achilles tendon, sedentary lifestyle, stiffness from long days of travel, sluggish energy, lack of balance, lack of self-confidence

Your feet are the foundation for standing, walking, dancing, playing sports, and more. Supple shins, flexible ankles, and responsive soles contribute directly to your ability to balance. Over time, the agility of your feet can diminish. When you limit your leg movements or wear less-than-optimal shoes, you limit circulation and flexibility, which can lead to tripping or falling. This heel-lift practice invites you to maintain Mountain Pose as you feel the uplift of energy and breath support, and your feet and lower legs become flexible and strong.

COMMON CONDITIONS ADDRESSED

- Balance issues
- Diminished lower-body circulation
- Plantar fasciitis
- Restricted toe flexibility
- Tight calves
- Uncoordinated breathing

PROPS NEEDED: CHAIR (OPTIONAL)

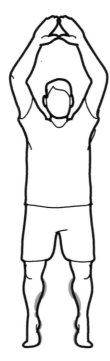

Coordinate the inhale as the arms sweep up, and exhale as the arms come down. Lift the heels just enough to feel the lower legs, calves, and feet stretch.

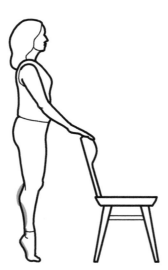

CHAIR VARIATION: Maintain Mountain Pose as the heels rise from the floor. Make sure the chair is on a stable surface.

1. Stand in Mountain Pose (see page 33).

2. Inhale and raise your arms out to the sides and over your head as though you're making angels in the snow. Exhale and bring your arms back to your sides. Repeat for 2 or 3 breaths.

3. While maintaining the upper body and breath movement, lift your heels off the floor. The space between the floor and your heels should be just enough to feel the stretch at the bottom of the feet, Achilles tendons, and calves. Maintain core engagement while breathing so you don't feel like you're toppling over.

4. Repeat this coordinated movement with the breath 8 to 10 times.

5. Pause in Mountain Pose, or keep your heels on the floor and lift your toes for a counterstretch.

TIP

Keep your eyes softly focused on the horizon.

MODIFICATION

If balance is a challenge, stand in front of a chair, placing your fingertips on the back for confidence and safety.

LEG STRETCH #1

PHYSICAL AREAS TARGETED: plantar fascia, Achilles tendon, gastrocnemius, hamstrings (see page 133)

BODY AND MIND AREAS RELIEVED: sore feet, tight ankles, stiff Achilles tendons, tight hips, tight calves, tight hamstrings, inflexibility of the lower body

Leg Stretch #1 helps lengthen the entire line of muscles and fascia (see page 21) in the back of the body. This strap-assisted stretch provides stimulation to the muscles and bones of the legs. If practiced while reclining, it's a safe forward fold for those with spinal conditions or osteoporosis. Beginners and longtime yogis alike can use this pose as a baseline for tracking increased flexibility with regular practice.

COMMON CONDITIONS ADDRESSED

- Back pain
- Plantar fasciitis
- Osteoporosis
- Sore feet

- Soreness from athletic activities
- Stiff lower body from a sedentary lifestyle
- Stress

PROPS NEEDED: YOGA STRAP, CHAIR (OPTIONAL)

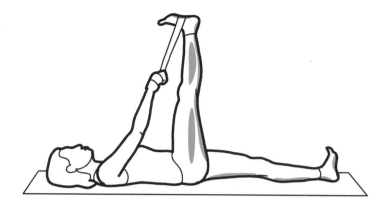

RECLINED VARIATION: Keep the lower leg active and the shoulders relaxed. Depending on your flexibility, the strapped leg may be either closer to your torso or farther away. Maintain a straight (not locked) knee to ensure that the hamstrings receive lengthening.

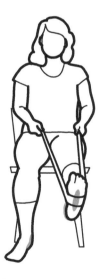

SEATED VARIATION: Maintain a strong spine and avoid rounding the spine toward the leg. If you are sitting on your tailbone, adjust the pelvis so it is neutral. Use the chair back if needed to maintain spinal integrity.

1. Recline on your back with both knees bent and heels hip distance apart.

2. Holding the strap in both hands, bring the right knee toward the chest and place the strap on the arch of the right foot.

3. Slowly straighten the right knee. Slide the left heel on the floor until the left leg is straight with your toes facing the sky. Make sure the left hip, knee, and ankle are in alignment, as though you were standing on the floor.

4. Move the strapped right foot into any position that keeps the right knee straight without overexerting it. If you are less flexible, the leg will move away from your upper body; if you are more flexible, the leg will move closer to the upper body.

5. After several breaths, expand the stretch by gently pressing the right heel toward the sky and pointing your toes toward your face. Your leg may not move, but you'll sense further opening. Maintain the pose for 5 to 10 breaths.

6. To come out of the pose, bend the right knee and release the strap. Rest for several breaths. Notice the difference between the two legs.

7. Repeat on the left side.

8. Continue this stretch with Leg Stretches #2 and #3 (see page 143) or Knees-to-Chest Pose (see page 111).

TIPS

- The strapped leg may shake a bit as you begin to gain flexibility. Over time, the shaking will subside. Keep the knee bent and the foot of your unstrapped leg on the floor if you are unable to straighten it.

- While holding the strap, keep the upper back and shoulder blades connected to the earth as the chest remains open for your breath.

- If you are very flexible, you may be able to grasp your big toe with your hand instead of using the strap.

• Experiment with placing the strap on the ball of the foot rather than the arch to vary the sensation. If you have plantar fasciitis, you may find improved relief with this placement.

• If you are unable to lie down on the floor, practice the seated variation. Sit with a strong spine toward the edge of the chair in seated Mountain Pose (see page 33). Lasso the strap on the left foot and keep the right foot connected to the earth. Maintain joint alignment of the hip, knee, and ankle of the strapped leg. After several breaths, expand the stretch by gently pressing the left heel forward and your toes toward you. Your leg may not move, but you'll sense further opening. Maintain the pose for 5 to 10 breaths, release the strap, and switch to the other side.

STAFF POSE WITH ANKLE CIRCLES

PHYSICAL AREAS TARGETED: plantar fascia, Achilles tendon, gastrocnemius, tibialis anterior, hamstrings, quadriceps (see page 133)

BODY AND MIND AREAS RELIEVED: sore feet, stiff Achilles tendon, stiff ankle joints, tight calves, decreased circulation, tight hamstrings

This deceptively simple series has myriad benefits. You can practice this anywhere, in any position, at any time. Maintaining mobility in your ankle joints contributes to increased flexibility in the joints as well as improved balance to prevent falls. As you employ the muscles above the feet to move the ankle joints, your lower-body circulation improves. The soleus is often referred to as "the second heart" because contracting the calves for these movements helps pump blood from the lower body back to the heart. From overactivity to underactivity, these movements are helpful for everyone.

COMMON CONDITIONS ADDRESSED

- Arthritis
- Difficulty walking
- Difficulty with balance
- Overuse and stress from athletic activities, such as tennis
- Plantar fasciitis
- Poor circulation from diabetes
- Recovery from uphill and downhill hikes
- Stiff lower body from a sedentary lifestyle

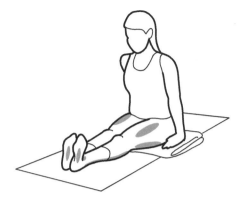

Place a blanket under your hips to
keep your spine from rounding.

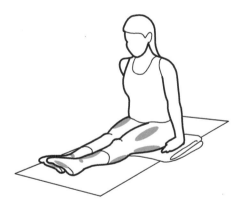

Feel the stretch in the front of your
ankles and shins as your toes point.

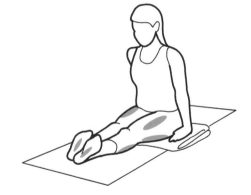

Feel the length in your ankles and
calves pumping blood as you move
your toes toward you.

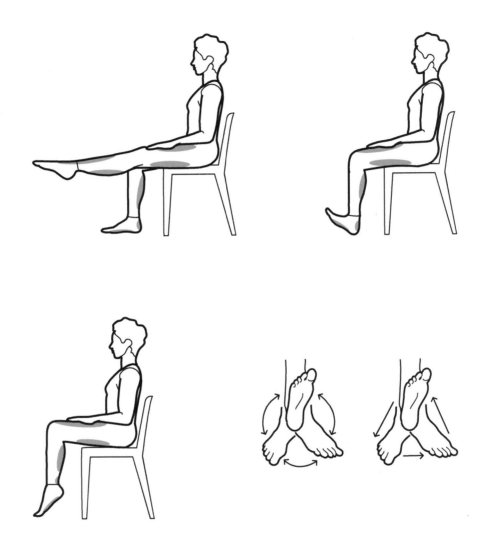

CHAIR VARIATIONS: Seated Staff Pose modifications with point and flex of ankles.

1. Position yourself in Staff Pose: Sit on the floor with your legs stretched out in front of you, approximately hip distance apart.

2. If your lower back is rounding and your shoulders are slumping, sit on 1 or 2 folded blankets.

3. Bring your fingertips or palms alongside your hips and continue to keep your shoulders relaxed and your chest open.

4. Repeat the following movements 10 to 20 times. As you warm up, increase the range of motion at the middle and end repetitions of each movement:

   · Point and flex the feet, simultaneously or one at a time. Imagine you are slowly pressing and then releasing the gas pedal of a car.

   · Rotate your ankles. Imagine there is a pen connected to your big toes and you are drawing circles in the air. Increase the circumference of each circle as your joints warm up.

   · Imagine your feet are like windshield wipers and let the toes drop away from and toward each other, keeping the heels on the ground.

   · Add any other creative movements. For example, pretend to catch a small ball with your toes and then spread your toes apart, or write your name in the air with your big toe.

5. Pause in Staff Pose and feel the warmth and circulation in your lower extremities.

TIPS

● Think of Staff Pose as a seated Mountain Pose (see page 33) in which you maintain the natural spinal curve and keep the pelvis neutral.

● Even though only your feet are moving, sense the pumping action into the shins, calves, and even the quadriceps and hamstrings.

● If you can maintain good posture, place your hands on your thighs above the knees and feel increased core muscle engagement.

MODIFICATION

If you are unable to sit on the floor, practice the same ankle movements in a chair. In the chair modification, you can keep both feet on the floor or straighten one leg and bring that foot off the floor.

HERO'S ANKLES

PHYSICAL AREAS TARGETED: plantar flexors: gastrocnemius, soleus, tibialis posterior, flexor digitorum longus, and flexor hallucis longus; dorsiflexors: tibialis anterior, extensor digitorum longus, and extensor hallucis longus

BODY AND MIND AREAS RELIEVED: tight shins, tight ankles, tight calves, shin splints, decreased circulation, lack of concentration

When you are standing in Mountain Pose or practicing balancing on one foot, your ankle joints are essentially positioned at a right angle. Consequently, the muscles in the shins can become tight and underused, affecting the ankle mobility needed for walking, balancing, and doing a host of athletic activities. My students are often surprised to discover the tightness at the front of their ankles when practicing this pose. The focus is stretching the shin muscles that move the ankles. Sit as high as needed on the props or use the chair or standing modification to relieve any pain or stress in the knee joints or quadriceps. Hero's Ankles variations are wonderful as stand-alone practices and as counterposes to the Half Forward Fold Pose (see page 169) and almost any other standing pose. Many yogis practice meditation in Hero's Ankles.

COMMON CONDITIONS ADDRESSED

- Difficulty walking
- Difficulty with balance
- Overuse and stress from athletic activities, such as tennis
- Poor circulation from diabetes
- Recovery from uphill and downhill hikes
- Stiff lower body from a sedentary lifestyle

PROPS NEEDED: BLANKET(S), BLOCK(S) , CHAIR (OPTIONAL)

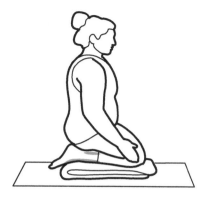

Stack as many blankets or blocks as needed for
comfort. Lift the spine and relax.

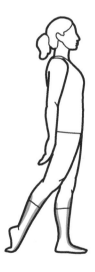

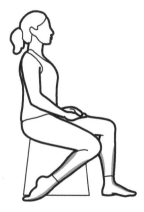

STANDING VARIATION:
Maintain Mountain Pose alignment
with the ribs over the hips.

SEATED VARIATION:
Maintain seated Mountain Pose. Make
sure the chair is stable. Optionally, you can
practice with both feet simultaneously.

1. Place a folded blanket on your mat, and a block or two on the blanket if needed.

2. Kneel so your toes are slightly off the blanket but your ankles and shins are supported.

3. Adjust your legs approximately hip distance apart and begin to sense your toes pointing straight back. Sit comfortably on the block or blanket.

4. Relax in the pose for 30 seconds to 1 minute. Keep breathing, and keep your shoulders relaxed.

5. To come out of the pose, lift the hips and remove the block.

6. Practice Staff Pose with Ankle Circles (see page 162) or any other ankle movement as a counterpose.

TIPS

- Do not force your hips or knees together or apart; everyone's body is different. Imagine they are pointing straight forward and parallel and adjust the width so you have no knee strain or hip pain.

- Over time, you may be able to sit directly on your heels rather than on the block; however, the goal is to safely stretch the ankles.

MODIFICATIONS

- Practice the seated or standing variation if you have knee or hip pain in the floor version, or other knee injuries or conditions.

- Seated variation: In seated Mountain Pose (see page 33), with an engaged core and relaxed shoulders, bring the top of your foot to the floor and point your toes back. Once you feel the ankle and shin stretch, breathe and feel the opening for 30 to 60 seconds. Repeat on the second side.

- Standing variation: From Mountain Pose, step one foot slightly behind you until you feel a stretch on the top of the foot and ankle. Maintain Mountain Pose and avoid leaning your torso forward or backward. Hold on to a chair or the wall for balance if needed.

HALF FORWARD FOLD

PHYSICAL AREAS TARGETED: gastrocnemius, soleus, hamstrings (see page 133), erector spinae (see page 69)

BODY AND MIND AREAS RELIEVED: tight hamstrings, tight ankles, tight calves, decreased circulation, lack of concentration

This pose is a safe variation of a traditional forward fold. Placing a rolled blanket under the heels helps the posture target the calves, hamstrings, and back line of the fascia and muscles. Without having to touch your toes, you can get stiffness relief in the posterior fascial line of the body (see page 21). You will also lengthen the spine for improved posture and practice engaging your breath to support the core muscles. This pose is safe for yogis who are pregnant or have osteoporosis.

COMMON CONDITIONS ADDRESSED

- Difficulty walking
- Overuse and stress from athletic activities, such as tennis
- Poor circulation from diabetes
- Recovery from uphill and downhill hikes
- Stiff lower body from a sedentary lifestyle
- Unsteady balance

PROPS NEEDED: BLANKET, WALL (OPTIONAL)

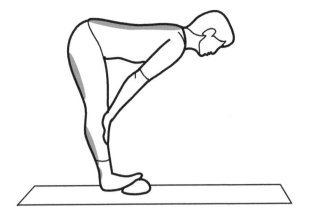

Keep your hips over your heels and length in the entire spine.

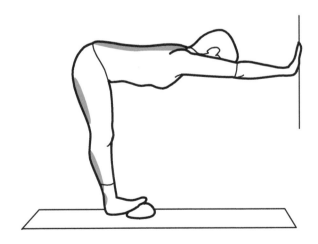

WALL VARIATION: Practice at a wall if balance is challenging.

1. Place a rolled blanket on your mat.

2. Stand in Mountain Pose (see page 33) in front of the blanket. One at a time, walk the balls of both feet onto the blanket so the heels are on the mat and the toes and balls of your feet are on the blanket.

3. Hinging at the hip, inhale, then exhale into a half forward fold, placing your fingertips anywhere on your legs that will allow you to keep your spine parallel to the floor.

4. Align your hips over your legs so you can maintain the natural curve of the spine.

5. Hold the pose for 5 to 10 breaths.

6. To release the pose, inhale and hinge back up to Mountain Pose, bending your knees slightly, if needed. Step off the blanket.

7. Stand in Mountain Pose, and if you'd like, follow up with Heel Lifts with Arm Waves Pose (see page 155).

TIP

Experiment with the thickness of the blanket. If your calves or hamstrings are extremely tight, you may need a short fold or you may not be able to use a blanket.

MODIFICATIONS

- If balance is a challenge, bring your mat and blanket to a wall. Stand facing the wall and take a practice forward fold to determine where to place the blanket. You should be in an L shape with your hands at the wall at shoulder height. Place the blanket where your feet are. Practice with your hands on the wall instead of your legs.

- If you are unable to stand, practice the ankle movements of the seated Staff Pose variation (see page 162).

Lower-Body Sequences

POSTURE FOCUS

PHYSICAL AREAS TARGETED

This sequence emphasizes many of the mind, body, and breath elements that contribute to postural poise: feet, ankles, breathing, mental presence and focus, and core awareness. In Staff Pose with Ankle Circles, you will become more attuned to core engagement and spinal integrity. Your feet are the base of your standing posture, and the ankle movements in Staff Pose help your ankles and feet become more supple. Any version of Tree Pose requires postural consciousness, and as you practice, you will often observe micro adjustments in the ankle joints as you improve balance. You'll complete the sequence in a Half Forward Fold, sensing a wonderful lengthening in the backs of the legs after Tree Pose.

Chest, Torso, and Back Muscles (see page 68)

- erector spinae

Hip, Gluteal, and Pelvic Muscles (see page 110)

- gluteus medius
- iliopsoas

Thigh and Knee Muscles (see page 133)

- adductor group
- hamstrings
- quadriceps
- tensor fasciae latae

Calf, Ankle, and Foot Muscles (see page 154)

- Achilles tendon
- gastrocnemius
- plantar fascia
- soleus
- tibialis anterior

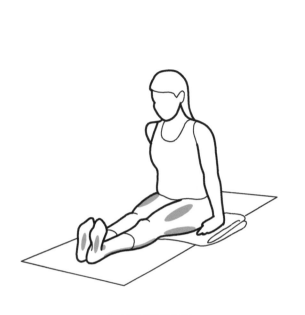

1. STAFF POSE

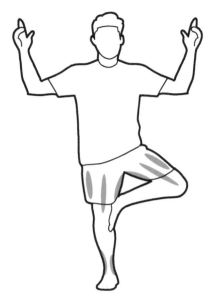

2. TREE POSE

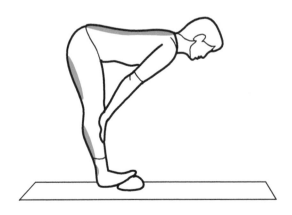

3. HALF FORWARD FOLD

1. Sit on the floor in Staff Pose and bring your ankles through the full range of movements as indicated on page 162. Remember to place as many blankets under your hips as needed to maintain good posture. Resume Staff Pose for several breaths, then make your way to standing.

2. Remove any blankets from the mat and stand in Mountain Pose (see page 33). Gaze at a point on the horizon and practice Tree Pose (see page 120), making sure to alternate the standing leg. Practice Tree Pose near a wall or chair, if needed, for confidence and safety. Notice the difference between the sides and return to Mountain Pose for several breaths.

3. Place a rolled blanket on your mat. From Mountain Pose, stand in front of the blanket. One at a time, walk the balls of both feet onto the blanket. Your heels will be on the mat and your toes and balls of your feet will be on the blanket. Practice Half Forward Fold (see page 169). Inhale and hinge back to Mountain Pose and observe a change in poise and posture.

TIP

Practice positive affirmations, such as "My posture is improving with practice" or "My breath supports my posture, and my posture supports my breath."

MODIFICATION

If you are rebuilding flexibility or strength, are recovering from an illness, are in the later stages of pregnancy, or have trouble balancing, modify the sequence by practicing each of these variations: seated Staff Pose with Ankle Circles, seated Tree Pose, and Half Forward Fold at the wall.

STRENGTH FOCUS

PHYSICAL AREAS TARGETED

This empowering sequence requires you to use your muscular strength, body weight, breath, and mental concentration to move between poses. The poses themselves lengthen, tone, and strengthen muscles with a primary focus on the lower body. By employing your body weight, you activate muscular capabilities and build bones. The standing poses in this sequence will increase your hip and leg strength. At the same time, you will develop flexibility, mental fortitude, awareness of upper- and lower-body coordination, focus, and a wonderful sense of empowerment.

Hip, Gluteal, and Pelvic Muscles (see page 110)

- gluteal muscles
- hip flexors
- psoas
- tensor fasciae latae

Thigh and Knee Muscles (see page 133)

- adductor group
- hamstrings
- quadriceps

Calf, Ankle, and Foot Muscles (see page 154)

- gastrocnemius
- soleus

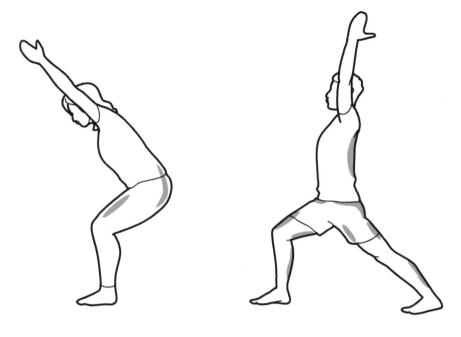

1. CHAIR POSE

2. WARRIOR I

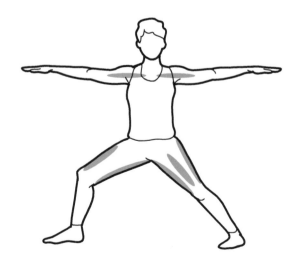

3. WARRIOR II

1. Beginning in Mountain Pose (see page 33) at the short end of the mat, practice Chair Pose (see page 117) for as many breaths as your current endurance allows. Place a block between your inner thighs if you want to increase awareness of the adductors.

2. Return to Mountain Pose.

3. Step back with one foot and take a wide stance, heels hip distance apart. Practice Warrior I (see page 126) on both sides.

4. After completing Warrior I, return to Mountain Pose for several breaths, then turn your body to face the long side of the mat. Step your feet as wide as you comfortably can and practice Warrior II (see page 137) on both sides.

5. Return to Mountain Pose and feel your physical and mental strength.

TIPS

- Begin by practicing each pose for 3 to 5 breaths and work up to 10 breaths, as your endurance allows.

- Be careful not to overestimate or underestimate your strength and endurance. Pay attention to your breathing and the sensations in your muscles. Breathe smoothly and steadily and engage your muscles without overly tensing. Practice positive affirmations, such as "I am becoming strong" or "I can do this."

MODIFICATION

If you are rebuilding strength, recovering from an illness, or in the later stages of pregnancy, modify the sequence by practicing each of these variations: High Chair Pose, Warrior I with chair or table support, and seated Warrior II. Start with 2 to 5 complete breaths in each pose.

FLEXIBILITY FOCUS

PHYSICAL AREAS TARGETED

You can practice this flexibility sequence to unwind after a fitness routine or long sedentary periods, or as its own soothing yoga series. The sequence addresses the muscles and fascia that surround the hips, legs, and knees from myriad directions. The leg stretch series lengthens, opens, and closes the hip joint and the muscles surrounding it while you're being supported on your back or in a chair. In Reclined Pigeon, you experience a stretch in the backs of the hips as the piriformis finds space. Finally, the front of the hips and thighs are lengthened with Dancer Pose.

Chest, Torso, and Back Muscles (see page 68)
- erector spinae
- quadratus lumborum

Hip, Gluteal, and Pelvic Muscles (see page 110)
- adductor group
- hip flexors
- pelvic floor
- piriformis and other deep rotators

Thigh and Knee Muscles (see page 133)
- hamstrings
- iliotibial band
- quadriceps
- tensor fasciae latae

Calf, Ankle, and Foot Muscles (see page 154)
- Achilles tendon
- gastrocnemius
- plantar fascia

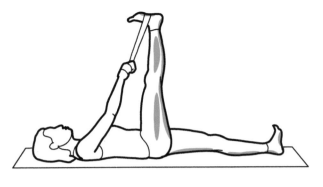

1. LEG STRETCH #1

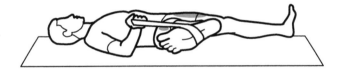

2. LEG STRETCH #2

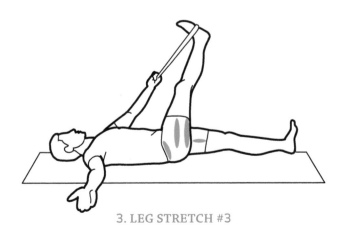

3. LEG STRETCH #3

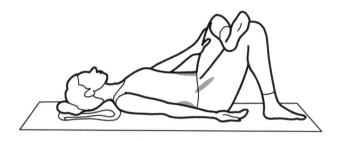

4. RECLINED PIGEON

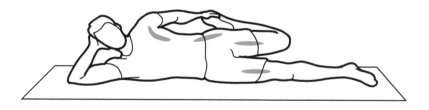

5. DANCER POSE

1. With a yoga strap nearby, recline on your back with both knees bent and your heels hip distance apart. Holding the strap with both hands bring the right knee toward the chest and place the strap on the arch of the right foot. Practice Leg Stretch #1 (see page 158), Leg Stretch #2, and Leg Stretch #3 (see page 143). Before placing the strap on your left leg, pause and feel the difference between the sides. Rest with your knees bent and your feet on the floor.

2. Hug the right knee into the chest. Rotating the leg at the hip, place the right ankle above the left knee. Remember to place a blanket under your head and neck if your chin is jutting toward the ceiling. Practice Reclined Pigeon Pose (see page 114) on both sides.

3. From Reclined Pigeon, practice Dancer Pose on the floor (see page 134), or if you wish, come to standing to practice the standing Dancer Pose.

TIP

Repeat positive affirmations, such as "I breathe freely as I become more flexible" or "Let go and unwind" as you practice.

MODIFICATION

If it is impractical to come to the floor or to stand, practice Leg Stretch #1 while seated on a chair, Leg Stretches #2 and #3 while seated on a chair, and seated Pigeon Pose.

A LITTLE BIT OF EVERYTHING

PHYSICAL AREAS TARGETED

Stretch, strengthen, and find a sense of yoga as a sanctuary from life's challenges as you practice this sequence. With this mini yoga class, you have the opportunity to bring your physical body to various accessible, empowering, and relaxing positions with three poses. Starting on your back and finding release in your hips and back, you will then practice both a standing stretch and a strengthening pose to fortify your day!

Chest, Torso, and Back Muscles (see pages 68–69)
- erector spinae
- quadratus lumborum

Hip, Gluteal, and Pelvic Muscles (see page 110)
- adductor group
- hip flexors
- pelvic floor

Thigh and Knee Muscles (see page 133)
- quadriceps

Calf, Ankle, and Foot Muscles (see page 154)
- Achilles tendon
- gastrocnemius
- plantar fascia
- soleus

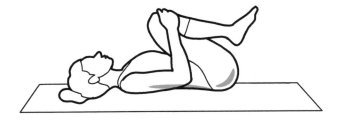

1. KNEES-TO-CHEST POSE

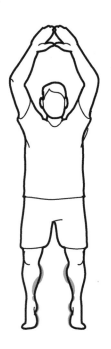

2. HEEL LIFTS WITH
ARM WAVES

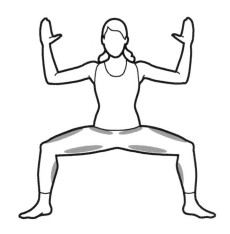

3. VICTORY/GODDESS SQUAT

1. Reclined on your mat, practice Knees-to-Chest Pose (see page 111), enjoying the lengthening and stretching of your lower back and hips for 5 to 10 breaths.

2. Make your way to standing in Mountain Pose (see page 33), facing the long side of the mat. Begin to uplift your energy in Heel Lifts with Arm Waves (see page 155) for 3 to 5 coordinated breaths. Pause in Mountain Pose, enjoying the vitality of your movements.

3. Now step your feet wide apart, facing the long side of the mat, and practice Victory/Goddess Squat (see page 123), statically or dynamically.

TIP

Practice supportive affirmations, such as "I heal my body and mind with my practice" and "Self-care is my priority."

MODIFICATION

If standing or balancing is a challenge, use these variations: seated Knees-to-Chest Pose, chair Heel Lifts, and seated Victory/Goddess Squat.

UNWIND AND DE-STRESS

PHYSICAL AREAS TARGETED

Practicing just three yin/restorative poses will help release your physical stress and mental tension. Allow gravity to unwind issues in your tissues (tight muscles, creaky joints, and sticky fascia), which are the result not only of repetitive postural habits but also of mental anxiety. We have discussed the stress-reducing effects of yoga on all layers of our being (koshas). The sequence below offers restorative positions that release hip, leg, and pelvic tension. You will have the opportunity to employ easy yogic breathing while practicing.

Chest, Torso, and Back Muscles (see pagess 68–69)
- intercostals
- obliques
- pectoralis

Hip, Gluteal, and Pelvic Muscles (see page 110)
- adductor group
- iliopsoas
- pelvic floor
- piriformis
- tensor fasciae latae

Thigh and Knee Muscles (see page 133)
- iliotibial tract
- quadriceps
- hamstrings

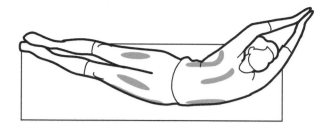

1. BANANA POSE

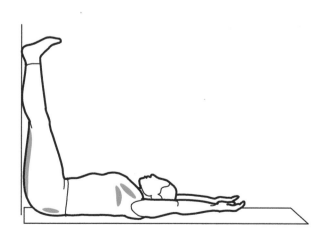

2. RECLINED BOUND ANKLE

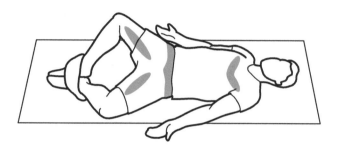

3. LEGS UP THE WALL POSE

1. Start with the short end of your mat next to the wall. Rest on your back with your legs together. Practice Banana Pose (see page 151) on both sides of the body for 2 to 4 minutes. Return to reclining on your back or take a full-body stretch in neutral with your arms over your head.

2. Making sure you have two blankets available, enjoy Reclined Bound Angle (see page 148) for 5 to 25 minutes. Using your hands, bring your knees together, stretch, and draw your knees to your chest.

3. Practice Legs-Up-the-Wall Pose (see page 129) for 5 to 20 minutes. With your hands braced on the floor behind you, lean your torso back slightly and swing your legs up the wall. Use props as necessary.

4. Notice the calming effects of this practice. Consider meditating in any comfortable position for 5 minutes or more.

TIPS

- A timer or stopwatch (check your phone for these tools, but make sure the ringer is off!) is handy when practicing yin and restorative poses. Set your timer for each pose, relax, and let the poses do their magic.

- Feel free to play unobtrusive, relaxing instrumental music when you are first practicing. Over time, you may not need it.

- To calm the mind and offer self-support, repeat to yourself for several breaths: "I deserve this time to unwind."

MODIFICATIONS

- If you are unable to come to the floor, practice Banana Pose and Reclined Bound Angle in bed or on a sofa that accommodates your body.

- Practice the legs-on-a-chair variation as an alternative to Legs-Up-the-Wall.

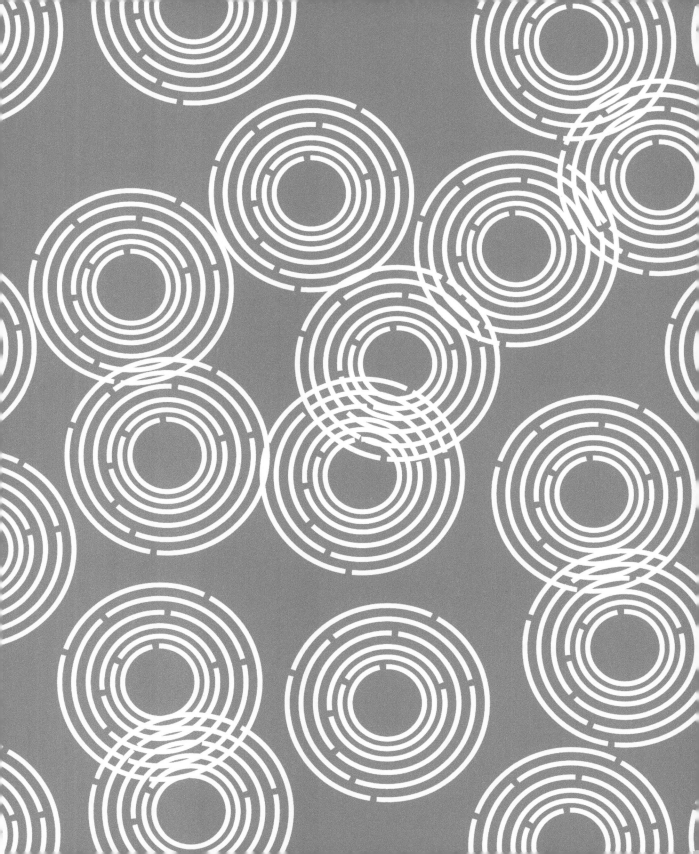

Resources

Bell, Baxter, and Nina Zolotow. *Yoga for Healthy Aging*. Boulder, CO: Shambhala, December 12, 2017. This comprehensive volume highlights yoga practices to age in a healthy manner.

Desikachar, T. K. V. *The Heart of Yoga: Developing a Personal Practice*. Rochester, VT: Inner Traditions, 1999. Breath-centered, accessible asanas and yoga philosophy from the master.

Howard, Leslie. *Pelvic Liberation: Using Yoga, Self-Inquiry, and Breath Awareness for Pelvic Health*. Leslie Howard Yoga, 2017. This book features yoga poses and breathing practices focused on female pelvic floor health.

Kaminoff, Leslie, and Amy Matthews. *Yoga Anatomy.* 2nd ed. Champaign, IL: Human Kinetics, 2012. This beautifully illustrated resource helps you learn more about anatomy, as well as how to use the breath in yoga poses.

Miller, Jill. *The Roll Model*. Las Vegas, NV: Victory Belt Publishing, 2014. This book features clear explanations of fascia, self–myofascial release, and how to use therapy balls to roll out tension.

Salzberg, Sharon. *Real Happiness: A 28-Day Program to Realize the Power of Meditation.* 2nd ed. New York: Workman Publishing, 2019. This guide to starting or restarting a meditation practice is from a down-to-earth and world-renowned teacher.

YinYoga.com. This dynamic website created by Bernie Clark encompasses all things yin yoga, including science, philosophy, poses, and discussions.

References

American Viniyoga Institute. "What Is Viniyoga?" Accessed January 22, 2020. viniyoga.com/about/what-is-viniyoga.

Ball, Elizabeth, Nur Shafina Muhammad Sharizan Emira, Franklin Genny, and Rogozinska Ewelina. "Does Mindfulness Meditation Improve Chronic Pain? A Systematic Review." *Current Opinion in Obstetrics & Gynecology* 29, no. 6 (December 2017): 359–366. doi: 10.1097/GCO.0000000000000417.

Basavaraddi, Ishwar V. "Yoga: Its Origin, History, and Development." Ministry of External Affairs, Government of India (April 23, 2015). mea.gov.in/in-focus -article.htm?25096/Yoga+Its+Origin+History+and+Development.

Benson, Herbert. *The Relaxation Response*. New York: Avon, 1976.

Biel, Andrew. *Trail Guide to the Body*. 3rd ed. Boulder, CO: Books of Discovery, 2005.

Clark, Bernie. *The Complete Guide to Yin Yoga: The Philosophy and Practice of Yin Yoga*. Rev. ed. Vancouver, BC: Wild Strawberry Publications, 2019.

Cole, Roger. "Relaxation: Physiology and Practice." From Relax and Renew teacher training materials with Dr. Judith Lasater. San Francisco, 2005.

Cramer, Holger, Petra Klose, Benno Brinkhaus, Andreas Michalsen, and Gustav J Dobos. "Effects of Yoga on Chronic Neck Pain: A Systematic Review and Meta-analysis." *Clinical Rehabilitation* 31, no. 11 (November 2017): 1457–1465. doi: 10.1177/0269215517698735.

Deslippe, Philip. "Yoga Landed in the U.S. Way Earlier Than You'd Think— and Fitness Was Not the Point." History (June 20, 2019). history.com/news/ yoga-vivekananda-america.

Duvall, Sarah Ellis. "Umbrella Breath." From Pregnancy and Postpartum Corrective Exercise specialist teacher training materials, online class, 2018.

Fishman, Loren, and Ellen Saltonstall. *Yoga for Osteoporosis: The Complete Guide.* New York: W. W. Norton & Company, 2010.

Haaz Moonaz, Steffany, Clifton O. Bingham III, Lawrence Wissow, and Susan J. Bartlett. "Yoga in Sedentary Adults with Arthritis: Effects of a Randomized Controlled Pragmatic Trial." *The Journal of Rheumatology* 42, no. 7 (July 2015): 1194–1202. doi: 10.3899/jrheum.141129. Epub 2015 Apr 1.

Hsu, Clarissa, William R. F. Phillips, Karen J. Sherman, Rene J. Hawkes, and Daniel C. Cherkin. "Healing in Primary Care: A Vision Shared by Patients, Nurses, and Clinical Staff." *Annals of Family Medicine* 6 (2008): 307–314. doi: 10.1370/afm.838.

Kaminoff, Leslie, and Amy Matthews. *Yoga Anatomy.* 2nd ed. Champaign, IL: Human Kinetics, 2012.

Kempton, Sally. "Getting to Know You: The 5 Koshas." *Yoga Journal.* yogajournal.com/yoga-101/getting-know. Last modified May 23, 2017.

Khalsa, Dharma Singh. *Yoga and Medical Meditation™ as Alzheimer's Prevention Medicine.* Alzheimer's Prevention Organization whitepaper, 2015. alzheimersprevention.org/downloadables/White_Paper.pdf.

Kundalini Yoga. "Fundamentals of Kundalini Yoga." Accessed January 22, 2020. www.kundaliniyoga.org/fundamentals.

Long, Ray. *The Key Muscles of Hatha Yoga.* 3rd ed. Baldwinsville, NY: Bandha Yoga Publications, 2006.

McCall, Timothy. "117 Health Conditions Helped by Yoga." Last modified June 2019. drmcall.com.

Myers, Thomas. *Anatomy Trains: Myofascial Meridians for Manual and Movement Therapists.* 2nd ed. London: Churchill Livingstone, 2009.

National Center for Complementary and Integrative Health. "Yoga Is One of the Top Ten Complementary Health Approaches." Last modified September 24, 2017. nccih.nih.gov/health/yoga-what-you-need-to-know.

National Institutes of Health. "More Adults and Children Are Using Yoga and Meditation." Last modified November 8, 2018. nih.gov/news-events/news-releases/more-adults-children-are-using-yoga-meditation.

Park, Seong-Hi, and Kuem Sun Han. "Blood Pressure Response to Meditation and Yoga: A Systematic Review and Meta-analysis." *The Journal of Alternative and Complementary Medicine* 23, no. 9 (September 2017): 685–695. doi: 10.1089/acm.2016.0234.

Pascoe, Michaela, David Thompson, and Chantal Ski. "Yoga, Mindfulness-Based Stress Reduction and Stress-Related Physiological Measures: A Meta-analysis." *Psychoneuroendocrinology*. 86 (December 2017): 152–168. doi: 10.1016/j.psyneuen.2017.08.008.

Pearson, Neil. "Integrating Pain Science, Education, Movement, and Yoga." In *Yoga and Science in Pain Care: Treating the Person in Pain*, edited by Neil Pearson, Shelly Prosko, and Marlysa Sullivan. London: Jessica Kingsley Publishers, 2019.

Ross, Alyson, and Sue Thomas. "The Health Benefits of Yoga and Exercise: A Review of Comparison Studies." *Journal of Alternative and Complementary Medicine* 16, no. 1 (January 2010): 3–12. doi: 10.1089/acm.2009.0044.

Saoji, Apar Avinash, B. R. Raghavendra, and N. K. Manjunath. "Effects of Yogic Breath Regulation: A Narrative Review of Scientific Evidence." *Journal of Ayurveda and Integrative Medicine* 10, no. 1 (January–March 2019): 50–58. doi: 10.1016/j.jaim.2017.07.008.

Saper, Robert B., Chelsey Lemaster, Anthony Delitto, Karen J. Sherman, Patricia M. Herman, Ekaterina Sadikova, Joel Stevens, et al. "Yoga, Physical Therapy, or Education for Chronic Low Back Pain: A Randomized Noninferiority Trial." *Annals of Internal Medicine* 167, no. 2 (2017): 85–94. doi: 10.7326/M16-2579.

Sengupta, Pallav. "Health Impacts of Yoga and Pranayama: A State-of-the-Art Review." *International Journal of Preventive Medicine* 3, no. 7 (July 2012): 444–458.

Slovik, Rolf. "Kosha Model." *Yoga International*. Accessed January 21, 2020.

yogainternational.com/article/view/kosha-model-overview.

Sohn, Emily. "The Heat of Hot Yoga Can Be Very Good—but Also Risky for Some People," *The Washington Post*, December 30, 2017. washingtonpost .com/national/health-science/the-heat-of-hot-yoga-can-be-very-good--but -also-risky-for-some-people/2017/12/29/150db00a-e1a3-11e7 -bbd0-9dfb2e37492a_story.html.

Stiles, Mukunda. *Structural Yoga Therapy: Adapting to the Individual*. Boston: Weiser Books, 2000.

Vaughn, Amy. *From the Vedas to Vinyasa: An Introduction to the History and Philosophy of Yoga*. Tucson, AZ: Open Lotus Publications, 2016.

Villemure, Chantal, Marta Ceko, Valerie A. Cotton, and Catherine Bushnell. "Insular Cortex Mediates Increased Pain Tolerance in Yoga Practitioners." *Cerebral Cortex* 24, no. 10 (October 2014): 2732–40. doi: 10.1093/cercor/bht124.

Yi-Hsueh Lu, Bernard Rosner, Gregory Chang, and Loren Fishman. "Twelve-Minute Daily Yoga Regimen Reverses Osteoporotic Bone Loss." *Topics in Geriatric Rehabilitation* 32, no. 2 (April 2016): 81–87. doi: 10.1097/ TGR.0000000000000085.

Yoga Alliance. "2016 Yoga in America Study Conducted by *Yoga Journal* and Yoga Alliance," January 13, 2016. yogaalliance.org/2016YogaInAmericaStudy.

Yoga International. "Ashtanga Q&A with Tim Miller." Accessed January 21, 2020. yogainternational.com/article/view/ashtanga-yoga-qa-with-tim-miller.

Pose Index

General Index

Acknowledgments

This book has been inspired by so many people in special and important ways. A special thank you to my managing editor, Claire Yee, for your ongoing respect, encouragement, and keen eye, and to my developmental editor, Debra DeFord-Minerva, for your confidence in this work.

I have abundant gratitude for the teachers with whom I have formally trained, particularly: Jill Miller, for setting high standards and "getting me" over the years from both near and far; Dr. Baxter Bell and Nina Zolotow, for your encouragement and philosophy of teaching yoga for healthy aging; Devi Daly, for helping me fall in love with yin yoga; and Linda Spackman, who helped me build a solid foundation for teaching yoga to pregnant women and plus-size bodies. Thank you to some of the many others I've trained and meditated with and who have wonderfully informed my practice and teaching, including: Sharon Salzberg, Dr. Judith Lasater, Dr. Roger Cole, Dr. Loren Fishman, Erich Schiffman, Menaka Desikachar, Dr. Shankaranarayana Jois, Dr. Sarah Duvall—and, of course, Tias Little.

I am always and forever grateful to my Tucson teachers and friends Chris Coniaris and Natasha Korshak, who have consistently and lovingly encouraged my offerings, and Jaimie Perkunas, a colleague and friend who provided the positivity and space for many of my specialized classes and workshops.

Thank you, with respect and love, to all my students, for the privilege of sharing my teachings and watching you become your own teachers. Special thanks to D. C.

Love is everything. Thank you to my family, who have supported me in my passion for yoga over all the years of practicing, teaching, and traveling, and in writing this book: Norm, Sam, Jesse, Ellie, Cheryl, Lynn, and Sadie.

About the Author

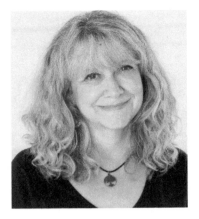

Bonnie Golden, MEd, E-RYT, specializes in teaching "yoga across the lifespan" with expertise in several yoga areas including pre-natal/postpartum, healthy aging, boomers, and beginners. She has guided thousands of students over many years in classes, workshops, and private sessions. Her students enjoy her accessible teaching style, which focuses on self-awareness, empowerment, calm, and fun! Bonnie's vast experience in teaching is fused with her love of lifelong learning, and she is honored to continually teach, educate, practice, write about, and study yoga and meditation. Her motto is "It's YOUR yoga"—and in public classes and private sessions, she encourages each student to honor their beautiful and unique mind/body/breath. In the early 2000s, after many years of teaching and sharing the tools of yoga for stress management, Bonnie formally qualified to teach yoga through international yoga master Tias Little (Prajna Yoga). At Prajna Yoga, she also successfully completed specialty training in prenatal yoga with Linda Spackman. She is a certified Yoga for Healthy Aging teacher, as well as a Pregnancy and Postpartum Corrective Exercise specialist. Further formal yoga training has included Relax and Renew training and several specializations of Yoga Tune Up. Bonnie has written for the Yoga Tune Up blog, *Yoga for Healthy Aging* blog, and is a published author on the subjects of self-esteem and psychological type (Myers-Briggs Type Indicator). She is a former college counseling faculty member. Learn more about her current offerings at YogaWithBonnie.com.